Clinical Virology

a guide for practitioners

George F. Winter, BSc, FIBMS

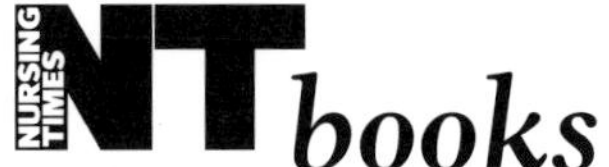

For my father and friend, George F. Winter (sen.)

First published 1999 by Nursing Times Books
Emap Healthcare Ltd, part of Emap Business Communications
Greater London House
Hampstead Road
London NW1 7EJ

Cover images courtesy of George F. Winter and Angus MacAulay
Cover design by Senate Design Ltd, London

Printed and bound in Great Britain by Thanet Press Ltd, Margate, Kent

British Library cataloguing in Publication Data
A catalogue record for this book is available from the British Library.

ISBN: 1 902499 65 4

Contents

Acknowledgements

This book would never have been possible without the help of a number of people.

I am extremely grateful to Emap Healthcare for publishing it, and to Alison Whyte who first gave me an opportunity to write for Nursing Times. Thanks also to Brian Booth and Martin Vousden at Nursing Times, who established the feasibility of the idea in the first place; to Simon Seljeflot and Jo Kemp, who helped co-ordinate the safe passage of the book into print; and to Penny Simmons who skilfully copy-edited the text.

Many thanks also to my colleagues Dr Heather A. Cubie for reading the initial drafts of the text and providing many invaluable comments; to Mrs Laura C. Kempton-Smith for reading the manuscript and advising on infection-control matters; to Mr Alastair J. Scott for his skill and dedication in executing the original drawings; and to Barbara Linton for providing the final artwork.

I am grateful to Faber & Faber Ltd. and to Peter and Claudia Ferguson-Smyth for permission to quote from Philip Larkin and George A. Ferguson respectively.

Finally, I would also like to thank Rita, for whose patience, support, editing skills and herbal teas I am very grateful.

Every effort has been made to ensure accuracy at all times. For any errors that remain, however, I alone am responsible.

Introduction

James Thurber said, 'it is better to know some of the questions than all of the answers.' During the course of their careers, many healthcare workers will have become acquainted with some of the questions commonly asked about viruses: what is a virus, how do viruses differ from other microbes, can virus infections be treated, how do viruses multiply? These, and other questions, are addressed here. Intended principally for nurses, this book aims to be a useful companion to those readers who do not intend to become virologists, but who wish to add some virological range to the focus of their individual discipline. Because of the sheer scope of the subject, this text is necessarily a work of selection and, as such, is not comprehensive, but tries to be comprehensible.

Why a book on viruses? There are two reasons. First, the demarcation between pure virology and medicine has become more blurred as our knowledge of events at a molecular level has increased. This means that a clear understanding of treatment regimes and diagnostic tests, for example, often depends on having a grasp of the nature of viruses and some of the basic molecular biological principles which apply to them.

The second reason is that it is perhaps time for a change of emphasis. From the early 1980s, the feeling that AIDS would become the virological *Zeitgeist* has quickly gathered a momentum which threatens to propel us towards the millennium believing that human immunodeficiency virus (HIV) is the only virus worthy of serious consideration. This ignores the fact that we are all, viruses included, part of a shifting landscape. So, it is timely for HIV not to be pushed out to the wings, but possibly nudged to the side a bit. Time to make way for those viruses that are making an impact now and are likely to continue to do so in the future. Some will always be with us, but poliomyelitis is going, measles should be going, and smallpox is gone. Yet through the revolving door of virology, here come the human herpesvirus types 6, 7 and 8; the expanding hepatitic realm of letters, to which hepatitis G is the latest addition; and the newly discovered transfusion-transmitted virus.

Part of the task of presenting a view of viruses is the choice of an appropriate format. There are literally hundreds of viruses which can infect humans, and these are classified on the basis of shared characteristics. The largest grouping is a family, denoted by the ending -*viridae*, and human viruses currently belong to 19 families. A common subdivision is the genus: for example, the influenzavirus genus belongs to the *Orthomyxoviridae* family. However, the oldest classification of viruses was based on the diseases they caused: convenient for clinicians, but unsatisfactory for virologists. In assuming a clinical bias for most readers, I chose a format which gives a general introduction to viruses, then focuses on specific sites of the body, and finally considers particular topics of interest from a general nursing perspective.

The first four chapters establish viruses as entities with characteristics which distinguish them from other microbes. Accordingly, when viruses are sought, specimen collection and laboratory diagnostic techniques must take account of the unique properties of these agents. The separation between the ward and the laboratory is less marked than before, with near-patient testing now a long-established feature of some diagnostic biochemical tests. This trend continues, with nursing staff becoming more directly involved in viral diagnosis. For example, the availability of near-patient testing kits for the rapid diagnosis of respiratory syncytial virus infection has resulted in their increased use in paediatric departments. This not only aids the clinical management of patients, but also fosters useful collaboration between ward and laboratory, and helps to develop a sense of being part of a wider team, an essential element in the clinical effectiveness agenda.

While considering selected systems of the body in Chapters 5–11, it is worth remembering that the same virus may appear in multiple sites, and the reader is encouraged to take an overall view of virus-cell interactions throughout the body. Historical perspectives to some topics are sometimes included at the expense of clinical signs and symptoms of disease, which can be found in standard texts. Chapter 8 includes a brief consideration of prions, a new biological concept which has gripped the public consciousness in the form of 'mad cow disease' and its new variant form which can infect humans.

Chapters 12–15 deal with particular topics of current interest. We consider how geography and human ecology determine some of the diverse thinking about HIV and AIDS. The wide application of chemotherapeutic options in the treatment of HIV, and other virus infections, has created a demand for more rapid diagnostic techniques which allow treatment to begin as early as possible. Antiviral therapy has contributed to the improved survival of transplant and other immunosuppressed patients, and these groups present the challenge of long-term virological surveillance, which, if it is to be effectively met, will demand ever closer liaison between medical, nursing and laboratory staff. One outcome of antiviral therapy already being seen with HIV is the problem of antiviral resistance; expect this to pose some infection-control challenges in the future. In the final chapter, oncogenic viruses are considered. The role of viruses in tumours is well established for some, and less so for others. For example, it is hoped that a future vaccine against certain human papillomaviruses can lead to a reduction in cervical cancer, while the role of the recently discovered human herpesvirus type 8 in Kaposi's sarcoma remains to be defined.

Given the modest aim of this book, there are bound to be omissions. However, many larger textbooks, and relevant review articles, are available for those wishing to fill gaps or supplement their reading.

1 The nature of viruses

Where the telescope ends, the microscope begins. Which of the two has the grander view?

Victor Hugo (1802–1885), *Saint-Denis*.

What's in a name?

Virus is an old Latin word meaning, 'Your guess is as good as mine'; a gentle hint that the occasional medical practitioner is sometimes not averse to hanging his stethoscope on a virus as a last diagnostic resort. Perhaps a virus is not so much a physical entity as a metaphysical abstraction. A face-saving solution; an elegant alternative to, 'I'm sorry, I've no idea'; a device for turning a fall into a dive. And we, the patients, so keen for the gap between ignorance and knowledge to be bridged, embrace the proffered virus unquestioningly. It might not *be* the truth, but it certainly has the *ring* of truth. And sometimes, it seems, that is enough.

'It's not responding to antibiotics … mmmm … it's probably a virus.'

'A virus. Oh, that's all right then.'

Well, sometimes it is – 'Viruses are just a fact of life, and you can't do much about them anyway' – and, as HIV, rabies and *Outbreak*, starring Dustin Hoffman, have shown, sometimes it is not.

The meaning of the word 'virus' has changed over the centuries and this might explain why viruses are sometimes confused with their larger cousins, the bacteria. For example, when newspapers report on cases of infectious disease, the evolution of a 'killer virus' to a 'deadly bacterium' can often be traced through the course of a single paragraph. In ancient Rome the word 'virus' was used to describe a *poison* of animal origin, and the diseases caused by these poisons were called 'virulent'. Today the word 'virus' denotes a distinct physical particle very different from bacteria, protozoa and fungi; indeed, these microbes, along with plants and animals, are themselves prone to viral infection. The AIDS era, recent experience with BSE, outbreaks of *E. coli 0157*, and antibiotic resistant bacteria have equipped the general public with a more sophisticated knowledge of things microbial than that which existed 20 years ago. As a result, there is an expectation that health professionals can augment this knowledge when asked to do so. Perhaps, therefore, it might help if we begin by putting viruses into some sort of historical context alongside their other microscopic chums.

Early days

The curtain was first raised on the microbiological landscape by Antony van Leeuwenhoek (1632–1723), a Dutch draper from Delft. While his contemporaries read Spinoza or cultivated Semper Augustus tulips, Antony was lens grinding: give him a lens and he would grind it for hours. He assembled his lenses into simple microscopes. These gave magnifications of up to about ×300, and he used them to examine bee stings, sheep hair, seeds and the like. One day he placed a drop of rainwater from a plant pot under his microscope. His eyes probably stood out on stalks *à la* Tom and Jerry, while a klaxon sounded, because in the rainwater a thousand creatures were capering, vibrant with life. He was the first person to see bacteria, protozoa, yeasts and fungi, but to van Leeuwenhoek they were all 'animalcules'. He recorded his observations and eventually sent them to the Royal Society of London, where they were sceptically received. It was in 1677, and only after the Royal Society had commissioned their own microscope to be made, that members saw, with their own eyes, that the cheese mite was no longer to be regarded as the smallest creature in Christendom (De Kruif, 1927). Van Leeuwenhoek continued his observations, in the course of which he became the first person to see spermatozoa under the microscope: presumably they were his. The faeces certainly were because in 1681, while suffering from diarrhoea, he put some of it under the microscope and became the first person to see *Giardia lamblia* (Collard, 1976). Microbiology was up and running.

In 1876 a German country doctor, Robert Koch, demonstrated that anthrax was caused by a type of bacteria called a bacillus. Six years later, he showed that the tubercle bacillus caused tuberculosis in humans. From these, and other, demonstrations of links between bacteria and disease came a series of criteria which had to be satisfied if a specific organism was to be the cause of a specific disease. They are called Koch's postulates and state that:

- the organism must be found in lesions of the disease
- the organism must be isolated in pure culture
- inoculating a pure culture of organisms into a new host will produce the disease
- the organism can be recovered from the lesions of the disease

By the end of the 19th century, microbiologists had the means of growing pure cultures of bacteria and fungi, microscopes to see them with, and Koch's postulates to apply when appropriate. As more bacteria were recognised as the agents responsible for many contagious diseases, they were referred to as the 'viruses' of disease. This was going to be a breeze, as it seemed that the presence of bacteria could soon be demonstrated for all infectious diseases. But it was soon clear that such confidence was wholly misplaced. Epidemics of smallpox, chickenpox, measles and influenza continued apace, and in addition, many plant and animal diseases occurred where no bacterial pathogen was implicated. Ironically, as early as 1885 Louis Pasteur had successfully used a vaccine against the virus causing rabies, without thinking that it might be an agent other than a sub-microscopic bacterium. As Pasteur might have said to Koch: 'Berlin … we have a problem.' Viruses were now about to emerge from the shadow of bacteriology and assert their own identity.

In 1879 Adolf Mayer began working in Holland with tobacco mosaic disease, which affects the leaves of the tobacco plant. He showed that the disease could be transmitted to healthy plants by the infected leaves of diseased plants, but failed to isolate a causative agent. Koch's postulates could not be satisfied. Following on from this, in 1892 Dmitri Ivanowski, a Russian botanist, passed the sap of infected tobacco leaves through a Chamberland filter that prevented the passage of bacteria, and found that it still retained its infectivity. Like Mayer, Ivanowski failed to grow the causative agent, again not satisfying Koch's postulates, but he had demonstrated the existence of a filterable virus, although he thought it was likely to be a toxin of some sort. Six years later, in van Leeuwenhoek's home town of Delft, Martinus Beijerinck, a botanist, extended Ivanowski's studies. He allowed filtered sap to sit for three months, then applied it to tobacco leaves where it produced disease; he discovered that alcohol and formalin, which killed other microbes, did not kill it, and he showed that it was not a toxin. But most important, he showed that the infectious filtered sap could only reproduce itself in living tissue. Between them, Mayer, Ivanowski and Beijerinck showed that tobacco mosaic disease was caused by an agent that was invisible under the light microscope, passed through filters which stopped bacteria, and multiplied only in living cells. Beijerinck originally called it a 'contagious living fluid', but realised that it must be a particle of some kind. Tobacco mosaic virus was the first 'filterable virus' to be discovered, and in 1939 became the first virus to be seen by electron microscopy (Fig 1.1). Much work was now undertaken, with the aim of demonstrating the filterability of those agents which had hitherto escaped detection by bacteriological methods.

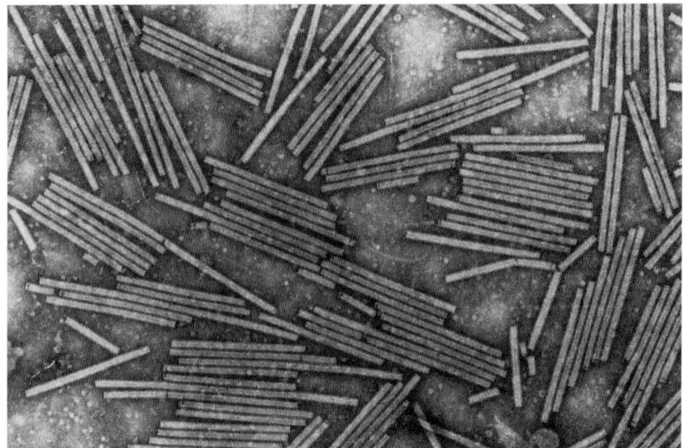

Fig 1.1 Tobacco mosaic virus in a leaf extract from an infected *Nicotiana clevelandii* plant. Magnification ×100,000

Source: Courtesy of Mr Ian M. Roberts, © Scottish Crop Research Institute, Dundee DD2 5DA

In 1898, the year when Beijerinck published his findings, the first filterable animal virus was discovered as the cause of foot-and-mouth disease of cattle, and in 1901 the first human filterable virus was discovered in Cuba as the cause of yellow fever. The first evidence that some viruses can cause cancer came in 1911 when Peyton Rous, working at the Rockefeller Institute, showed that a tumour-producing agent (he did not use the word *virus*) could be transmitted to chickens in a cell-free filtrate; today it is known as Rous sarcoma virus. Having only recently emerged from the shadow of bacteria, more viruses were now being discovered, much to the bemusement of bacteriologists. Imagine their dismay therefore when *bacteria eaters* came along. In 1915–17, Twort and d'Herelle, working independently in London and Paris respectively, discovered viruses that infect bacteria. D'Herelle called them bacteriophages, and their subsequent study has made a major contribution to modern biology. Over the next 20 years the fundamental properties of these viruses were investigated. In the 1940s detailed study of bacteriophages, particularly those infecting *Escherichia coli*, allowed rapid progress to be made in molecular genetics. In 1948 Sanford et al described the successful culture of single animal cells. In the same year, at Harvard Medical School, John Enders and co-workers discovered that poliovirus could grow in cell cultures of non-nervous tissue, a discovery which won them a Nobel prize in 1954. This reduced, at a stroke, the role of monkeys in poliomyelitis research, and gave impetus to the search for a vaccine. In 1955 Jonas Salk made the first effective poliomyelitis vaccine. Meanwhile, phage studies in the 1950s played an important role in leading up to the discovery that deoxyribonucleic acid (DNA) was the main repository of genetic information. Virology, as a distinct laboratory science, was established.

Unlike bacteria, which can be grown on a cell-free medium to produce colonies visible to the naked eye, viruses cannot multiply outside living cells. They are intracellular parasites, but, uniquely, their parasitism is at the genetic level. Viruses simply hijack the host cell's machinery and use it to express viral genes rather than host genes. The components specified by the viral genes are manufactured, assembled into viruses, and these are released from the host cell. The damage to the host cell is often, but not always, fatal. Viruses are unique in their simplicity of composition and their means of replication.

SIZE

Viruses are measured in nanometres (nm). One nm = 10^{-9} metres. They are all small, but with large variations in size (Fig 1.2). For example, the brick-shaped poxviruses are the largest animal viruses and can measure 300nm in length, whereas polioviruses are 18–30nm in diameter. Somebody once said that a virus penetrating broken skin is like throwing a golf ball into the Grand Canyon. If it was a bacterium, you would be lobbing in a large fridge-freezer.

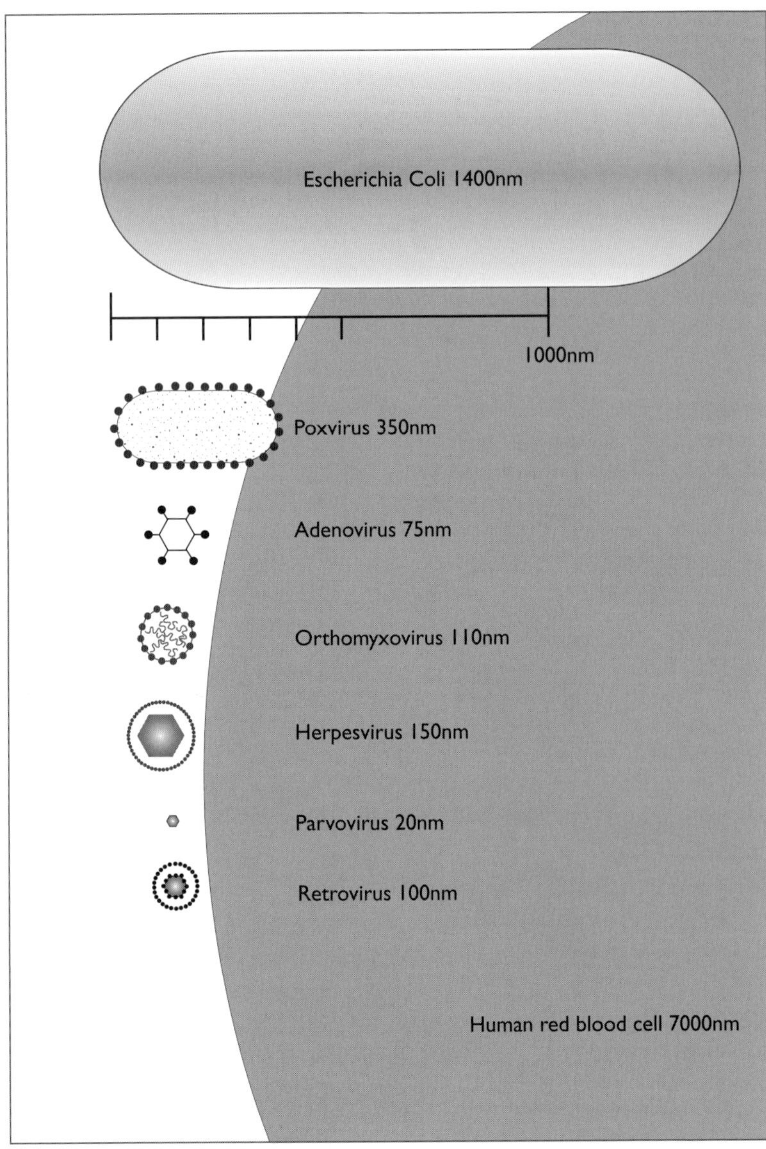

Fig 1.2 Comparative sizes of viruses, bacteria and human red blood cells
Source: Alastair J. Scott

Structure

A complete virus particle, or virion, consists of genetic information surrounded by a protective protein coat. The genetic information is contained in the virus nucleic acid or genome. The protein coat is called a capsid and is composed of sub-units called capsomeres. The combination of nucleic acid and capsid is called the nucleocapsid. Many viruses are surrounded by an envelope, made of lipids and proteins, which is largely derived from the outer membrane of the host cell (Fig 1.3). With certain viruses, such as measles virus and influenzavirus, glycoproteins project from the surface and are seen as well-defined spikes.

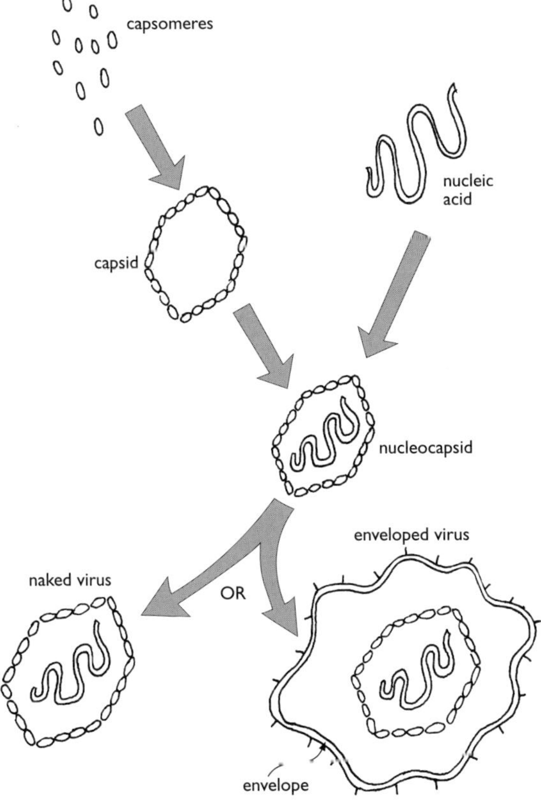

Fig 1.3 Virus structure
Source: Alastair J. Scott

The shapes of virions usually conform to one of three types of symmetry:

- *Cubic* – The protein shell is an icosahedron with the nucleic acid inside. (An icosahedron is a regular polyhedron with 20 triangular faces and 12 corners.) For example, adenoviruses (Fig 1.4) and polioviruses have icosahedral symmetry, whereas herpes viruses are icosahedrons surrounded by an envelope.

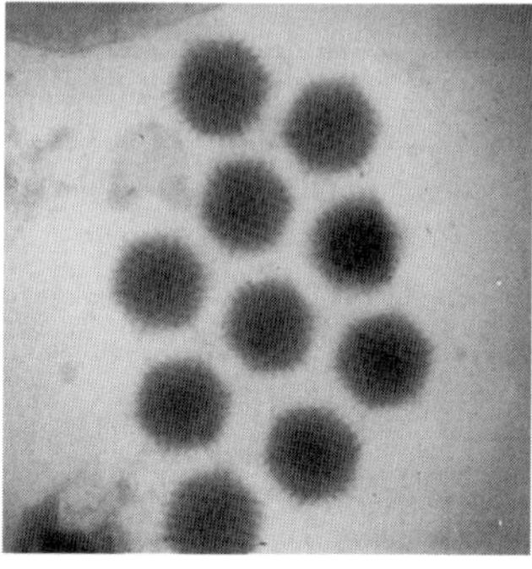

Fig 1.4 Icosahedral symmetry. Adenovirus in faeces from a child with acute diarrhoea and vomiting
Source: Courtesy of Dr W. D. Cubitt, Great Ormond Street Hospital for Children NHS Trust, London WC1N 3JH

- *Helical* – The proteins of the nucleocapsid assume a helical shape, herringbone-like, surrounding the nucleic acid core. The nucleocapsid is usually coiled within an envelope: for example, the viruses of measles, influenza and parainfluenza (Fig 1.5).

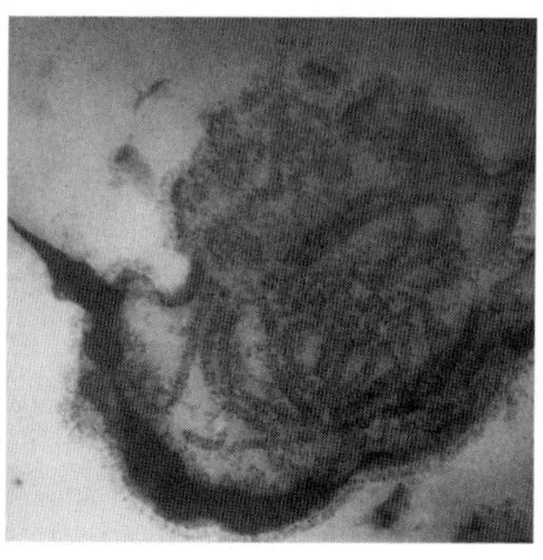

Fig 1.5 Helical symmetry. Parainfluenza virus type 3 isolated from a throat swab. Note herringbone-like appearance of nucleocapsids
Source: Courtesy of Dr W. D. Cubitt, Great Ormond Street Hospital for Children NHS Trust, London WC1N 3JH

- *Complex* – Poxviruses, for example, are brick-shaped or ovoid. They have several lipid-protein coats surrounding the nucleic acid, but conforming neither to cubic nor helical symmetry (Fig 1.6).

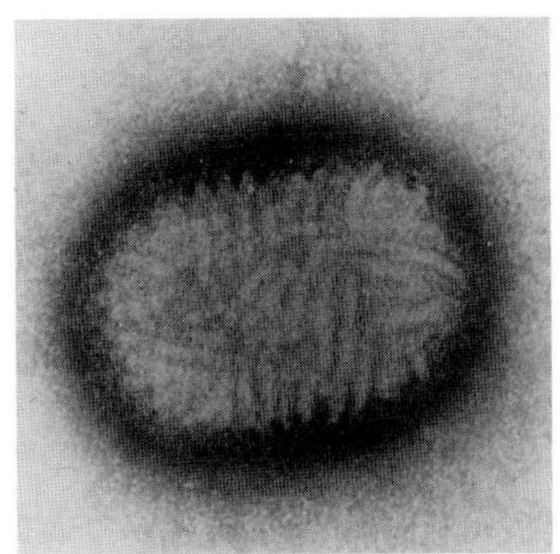

Fig 1.6 Complex symmetry. Molluscum contagiosum, a poxvirus, from a skin lesion
Source: Courtesy of Dr W. D. Cubitt, Great Ormond Street Hospital for Children NHS Trust, London WC1N 3JH

EFFECT OF CHEMICAL AND PHYSICAL AGENTS

Some viruses are poor survivors outside the host cell, whereas others can be as tough as old boots. The sensitivity of viruses to physical and chemical agents is a contributing factor to how effectively they can spread. For example, herpesviruses have envelopes which contain lipid, and are therefore sensitive to ether and other lipid solvents. The envelope is vital in gaining entry to cells, but if it becomes damaged, the virus will be inactivated. In contrast, rotaviruses, which have no envelope, are resistant to treatment with lipid solvents. Contact with contaminated surfaces is an important means of rotavirus transmission, and it was shown (Lloyd-Evans et al, 1986) that while certain chemical combinations inactivated rotavirus particles, many alcohol- and phenol-based conventional disinfectants were ineffective. This fact gains importance when we consider that at the peak of diarrhoea, there can be up to 100,000 million viruses in 1ml of faeces (Desselberger, 1996).

Enteroviruses, such as poliovirus, are identical in size and shape to rhinoviruses, which cause colds; indeed, they belong to the same virus family, sharing many other characteristics (Andrewes, 1989). However, they are distinguished by their relative sensitivities to pH. As enteroviruses can be found in the gut, it is not surprising that they can survive in acidic conditions, and their stability is unaffected at pH 3. In contrast, rhinoviruses, which are usually confined to the upper respiratory tract, lose their infectivity at pH 3. This difference in pH sensitivity is the basis for the acid lability test which can be performed in the laboratory to distinguish between an enterovirus and a rhinovirus.

Cultivation

Initially, the main source of living cells for growing viruses was the laboratory animal. For example, in 1933 Andrewes, Laidlaw and Smith successfully used ferrets to isolate, for the first time, the virus which caused influenza in humans. However, ferrets, primates and guinea pigs are not user-friendly, and more manageable vehicles for the growth of viruses had to be sought. Although attempts at cell culture were made throughout the 1920s, the lack of antibiotics to control bacterial contamination was a big obstacle to progress. In the early 1930s the embryonated hen's egg began to be used. Less vicious than a ferret, it was useful for growing a range of viruses. For example, influenzavirus could be grown in the amniotic and allantoic cavities of the egg, while smallpox and herpes simplex viruses could be grown on the chorioallantoic membrane, producing characteristic spots or pocks on the surface. With the availability of penicillin and streptomycin in the 1940s bacterial contamination could be controlled, and the subsequent development of cell-culture techniques soon led to a rapid expansion in virology, with the 1950s seeing the discovery of many new viruses.

However, it should be noted that not all viruses can be propagated in cell culture. For instance, rotavirus, human immunodeficiency virus (HIV), the hepatitis viruses and the human papillomaviruses do not grow in routine cell cultures. Nevertheless, most diagnostic virus laboratories have a cell-culture facility dedicated to the production of single layers of cells inside glass test-tubes. When cells are infected with a virus, it grows inside the cells and eventually kills them. This cytopathic effect (CPE) of the virus on the cell can be observed with an ordinary light microscope and test-tubes inoculated with specimens from patients can be examined routinely for CPE.

Although most routine cell culture uses cells grown on glass or plastic surfaces, the study of HIV has added impetus to the development of methods of long-term lymphocyte culture in liquid suspensions. The recent discovery of a new human herpesvirus was a direct result of the application of such methods (Braun et al, 1997). While recent developments in molecular techniques might place less reliance on cell culture as a diagnostic aid in the future, it is presently an important requirement for routine diagnostic work, and we could reasonably expect it to remain an integral part of any large diagnostic virus laboratory.

References

Andrewes, C. (1989) Picornaviruses. In: Porterfield, J. S. (ed.) *Viruses of Vertebrates*. London: Baillière Tindall.

Braun, D. K., Dominguez, G., Pellett, P. E. (1997) Human herpes virus 6. *Clinical Microbiology Reviews*; 10: 3, 521–567.

Collard, P. (1976) *The Development of Microbiology*. Cambridge: Cambridge University Press, p. 171.

De Kruif, P. (1927) *Microbe Hunters*. London: Jonathan Cape.

Desselberger, U. (1996) Classical and molecular techniques for the diagnosis of viral gastroenteritis. *Clinical and Diagnostic Virology*; 5: 101–109.

Lloyd-Evans, N., Springthorpe, V. S., Sattar, S. A. (1986) Chemical disinfection of human rotavirus contaminated inanimate surfaces. *Journal of Hygiene*; 97: 163–173.

Sanford, K. K, Earle, W. R, Likely, G. D. (1948) The growth *in vitro* of single isolated tissue cells. *Journal of National Cancer Institute*; 23: 1035–1069.

2 Cells and viruses

Shall I, like a hermit, dwell
On a rock or in a cell?

Sir Walter Ralegh (1552–1618), 'Poem'.

CELLS

In biology the cell is the basic unit of living matter, a microscopic Sistine Chapel where architecture and artistry fuse to resonate as a celebration of life itself. So, before it meets with some virological vandalism, it is fitting to have a short tour of the scene-of-the-crime-to-be, and a word from our sponsor – the uninfected cell (Fig 2.1).

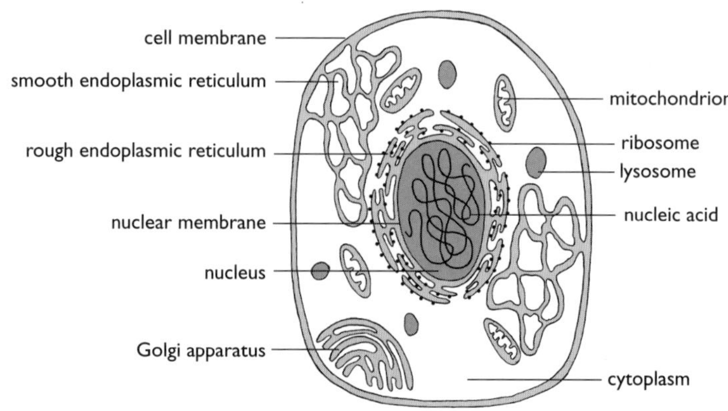

Fig 2.1 A 'typical' animal cell
Source: Alastair J. Scott

Although cells perform a diversity of tasks, they share many common features in their structure and function. In a 'typical' animal cell the genetic information is contained in the nucleus, where the chromosomal deoxyribonucleic acid (DNA) is held. The nucleus communicates with the rest of the cell, the cytoplasm, through pores in the nuclear membrane surrounding the nucleus. The endoplasmic reticulum (ER) is a protein factory, but also contains enzymes involved in the production of lipids. Some regions of the ER are studded with ribosomes, which are sites of protein synthesis. The Golgi apparatus is associated with the ER, and helps sort out which proteins are secreted from the cell and which are retained. The mitochondria are involved in energy production, and

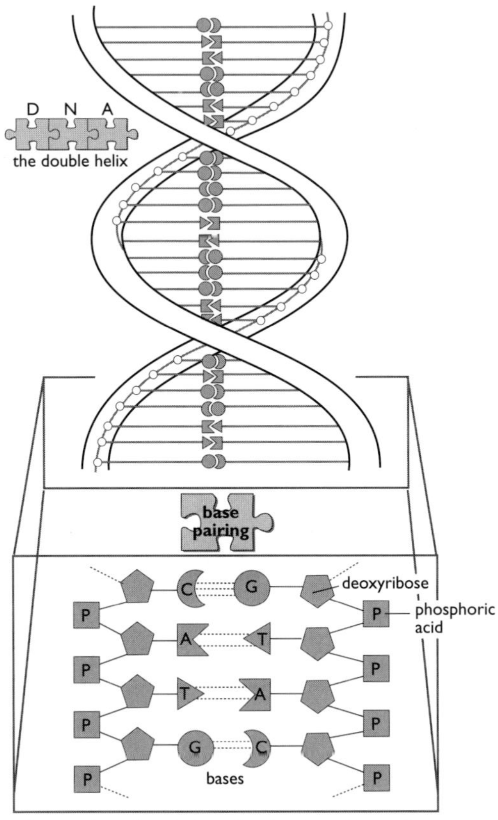

Fig 2.2 The structure of DNA
Source: Alastair J. Scott

lysosomes contain enzymes which help in the digestion of materials brought in from outside. The cell is bounded by a cell membrane which is a lipid bilayer, sandwiched between two protein layers.

The molecular basis for the information we call genes is DNA, which consists of two polynucleotide strands wound around each other to form a double helix. In DNA a single nucleotide is made from phosphoric acid, a sugar called deoxyribose and a base (Fig 2.2). The bases project inwards from each strand and are of four types: adenine (A), guanine (G), cytosine (C) and thymine (T). The size and shape of the bases are such that only A can fit together with T, and only G can fit together with C. They can 'recognise' each other, and are called complementary base pairs. Genetic information is passed from one cell to another because DNA can unzip its double helix, and replicate itself by incorporating new bases into positions complementary to the existing bases on each of the two single exposed strands (Fig 2.3). A gene is a length of DNA which codes for a particular protein. From the base alphabet of four letters (A, G, C and T), a series of

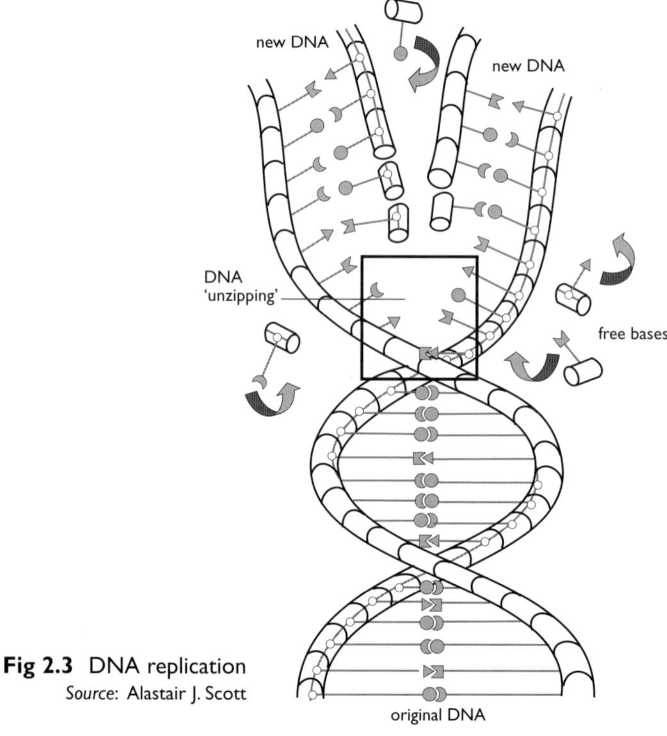

Fig 2.3 DNA replication
Source: Alastair J. Scott

three-letter words, or codons, is spelt out by the gene. The genetic code, which is used by almost every living organism from *E. coli* to man, translates the codons into a chain of amino acids, which will become a protein. It is the order in which the amino acids are linked which determines the protein that is made. As there are 20 different amino acids it is possible to make many different proteins: from hair to hormones to haemoglobin. Thus, *E. coli* has about 3,000 different kinds of protein, whereas man has around five million (Lehninger, 1972).

Inside a living cell, molecules are constantly being broken down or built up, with thousands of reactions occurring simultaneously. There is a group of proteins called enzymes whose function is to speed up the chemical reactions occurring in the cell. Every cellular process is governed by an enzyme that is generally involved in a single specific reaction. For example, when DNA replicates the operation is speeded up by the presence of the enzyme DNA polymerase.

In 1956 Francis Crick introduced the 'central dogma' of molecular biology which dictates that the flow of information is from DNA to protein. DNA is contained in the cell nucleus, yet proteins are made in the cell cytoplasm. There must be some sort of intermediary, or messenger, to take the message from the DNA in the nucleus into the cytoplasm. It is called messenger ribonucleic acid (mRNA), and is similar to DNA in that it is made up of a sequence of bases linked to form a chain. However, the sugar molecule in RNA is ribose rather than deoxyribose, and in RNA the chain is not double-stranded, nor is it helical; it is linear. In RNA thymine (T) is replaced by uracil (U). This means that when A appears on the DNA strand, U rather than T will appear on the corresponding mRNA strand. Copying the gene into a strand of mRNA is called transcription, and is catalysed by an enzyme called RNA polymerase. Not all of the codons code for amino acids; three of them are 'stop' messages which signal the end of the message. When the RNA polymerase reaches a stop codon the mRNA strand is completed, and it then moves from the nucleus to the cytoplasm, where the message is translated into protein. For example, the codon CAA on a gene will be transcribed into GUU on the mRNA which will be translated into the amino acid valine; this process is mediated by another type of RNA called transfer RNA. Translation occurs on the ribosomes, located in the ER in the cytoplasm, and through which the mRNA moves like tape through a tape-recorder (Fig 2.4). After our brief tour of the basic machinery of the uninfected cell, let us see what happens when a virus comes along.

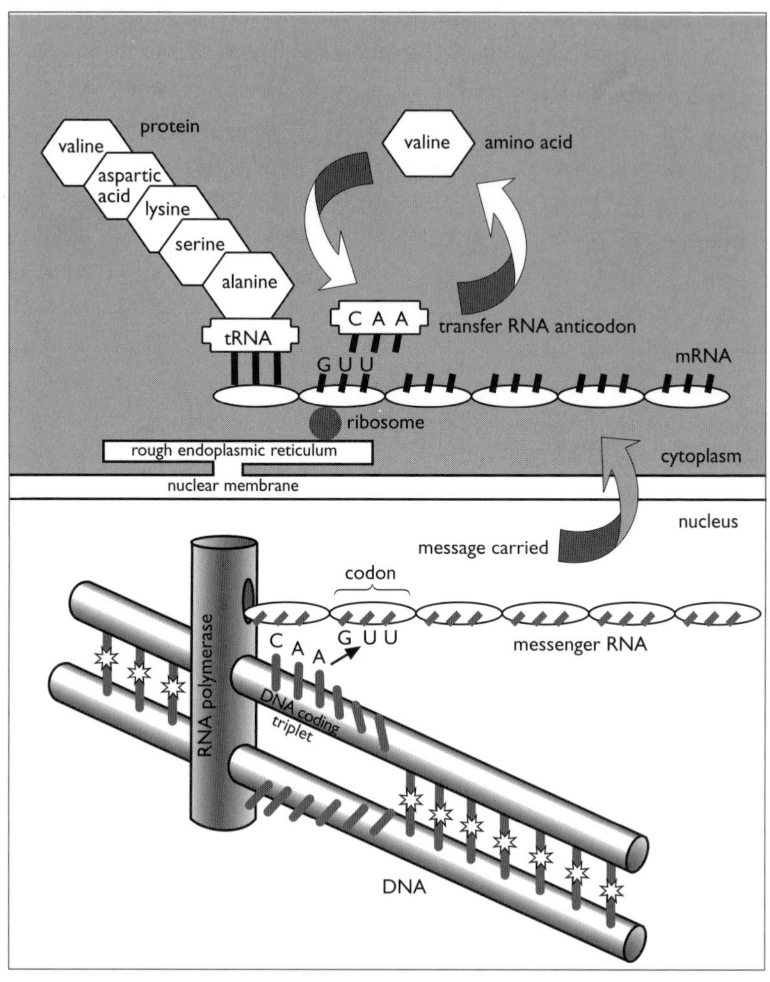

Fig 2.4 From DNA to protein
Source: Alastair J. Scott

VIRUSES

The entry of virus into the cell consists of:

- *Attachment or Adsorption* There are specific receptors on the surface of the cell to which the virus attaches. If these receptors are absent, infection will not occur. For example, influenzaviruses attach to mucoprotein receptors, polioviruses attach to lipoprotein receptors, and the human immunodeficiency virus (HIV) attaches to CD4 receptors on T4 lymphocytes. It is estimated that for a given virus, there are at least 100,000 receptor sites on each susceptible cell (Brooks et al, 1991).

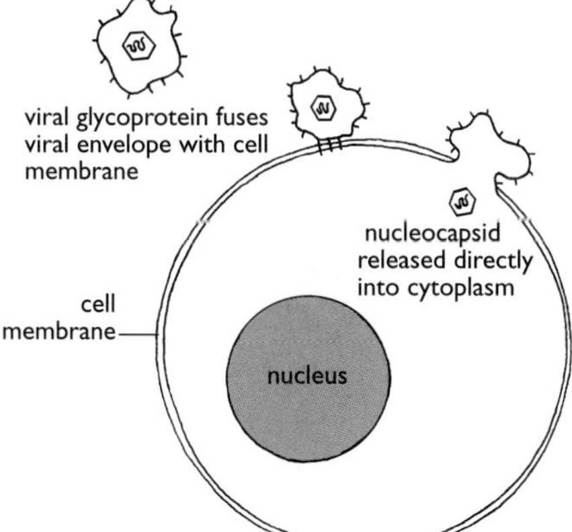

Fig 2.5 Virus entry into a cell by fusion
Source: Alastair J. Scott

- *Entry or Penetration* Shortly after adsorption the virus is taken into the cell. With enveloped viruses, such as herpes simplex virus or influenzavirus, the envelope fuses with the host cell membrane (Fig 2.5). Paramyxoviruses, such as measles virus, have a fusion protein which mediates in the fusion of the viral envelope with the host cell membrane, and is also involved in the spread of virus from cell to cell. Naked virions, such as enteroviruses, penetrate through the cell membrane directly into the cell. In addition, viruses may be taken into cells by viropexis (Fig 2.6). There are areas of the cell membrane where the protein clathrin is found. When the virus attaches here, the cell membrane inverts and forms a vacuole around the virus which is taken into the cell.

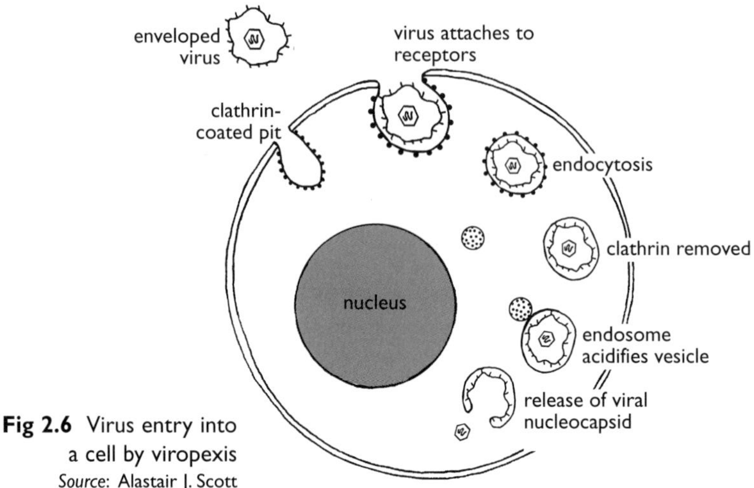

Fig 2.6 Virus entry into a cell by viropexis
Source: Alastair J. Scott

- *Uncoating* This consists of the removal of the protein coat or capsid by the action of cellular enzymes contained in the host cell, and it exposes the viral nucleic acid, or genome, allowing replication to begin prior to the assembly of virus particles.
- *Replication and Assembly* Kenneth M. Smith (1963) wrote: 'In considering how viruses multiply or replicate themselves it is best to avoid any comparison with the growth of an organism – a general picture of biosynthesis emerges, an assembly rather than a multiplication.'

We have seen the importance of mRNA in cells by the way it provides the link between the transcription of the genes encoded in DNA and their translation into defined sequences of amino acids which become proteins. Similarly with viruses, specific mRNA molecules must be transcribed from viral nucleic acid if the genetic information is to be expressed and duplicated. For the virus to survive, it is essential that it produces viral mRNA.

There are RNA-containing viruses and there are DNA-containing viruses. Although different pathways are used, the viruses have a common 'aim', which is the production of mRNA that can be translated into viral coat proteins and other proteins required for the replication of viral nucleic acid.

With DNA viruses, two types of virus mRNA are produced. Adenoviruses and herpes simplex viruses hijack a host cell RNA polymerase to make early mRNA. This is translated into the enzymes needed to help make virus DNA. For example, during adenovirus replication, at least 20 early proteins involved in the production of viral DNA are made. Once viral DNA has been made, a second type of mRNA – late mRNA – is transcribed from new virus DNA, and is translated into structural proteins which protect the nucleic acid. Once the protein coats (capsids) are made, they move from the cytoplasm into the nucleus where they combine with virus DNA. In the case of adenoviruses, stable infectious viruses now accumulate in the cell which will eventually burst. With herpes simplex, the virus acquires its envelope as it buds through the nuclear membrane of the cell (Fig 2.7).

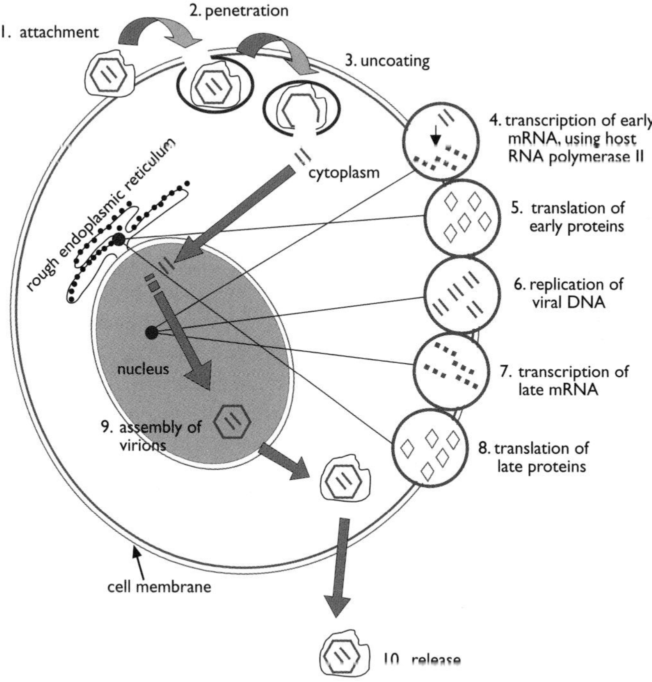

Fig 2.7 DNA virus replication using herpes simplex virus as an example
Source: Alastair J. Scott

RNA viruses can be divided into two groups. In the first group, when RNA viruses infect a host cell, the nucleic acid serves not only as the source of genetic information, but also as its own mRNA; such viruses are 'positive-stranded' (Fig 2.8). For example, when poliovirus RNA is exposed inside the cell, it is translated into a series of proteins. One of these proteins is an RNA polymerase, which is needed to make more viral RNA. In the second group, which includes influenza, measles and mumps viruses, the infecting RNA does not act as mRNA, and instead has first to be transcribed into a complementary strand of mRNA; such viruses are 'negative-stranded' (Fig 2.9). This transcription uses an RNA polymerase which is already present inside the infecting virus particle. The virus has to carry its own RNA polymerase to enable it to get to the mRNA stage.

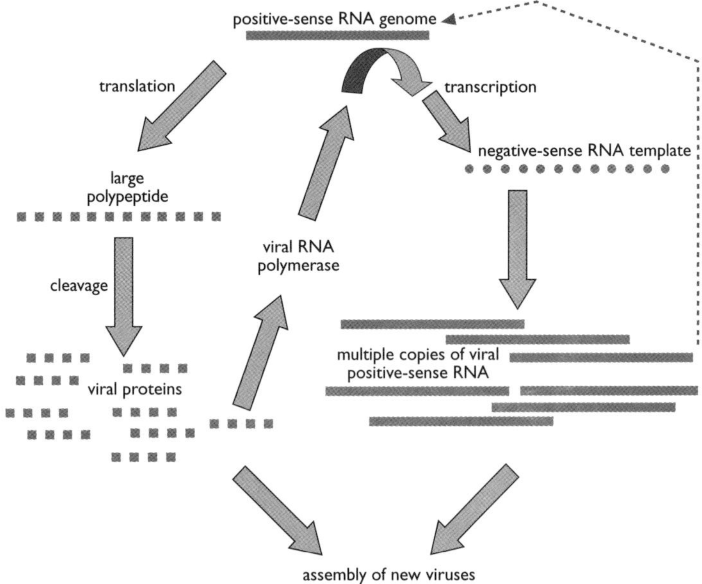

Fig 2.8 Replication of a 'positive-stranded' RNA virus
Source: Alastair J. Scott

This contrasts with poliovirus, whose RNA is already in messenger form and simply has its RNA polymerase translated when it is in the host cell. With both groups of RNA viruses, replication and assembly occur in the cytoplasm, except for influenzavirus which has a nuclear phase. Lastly, there is one group of RNA viruses, the retroviruses, which deserves special attention.

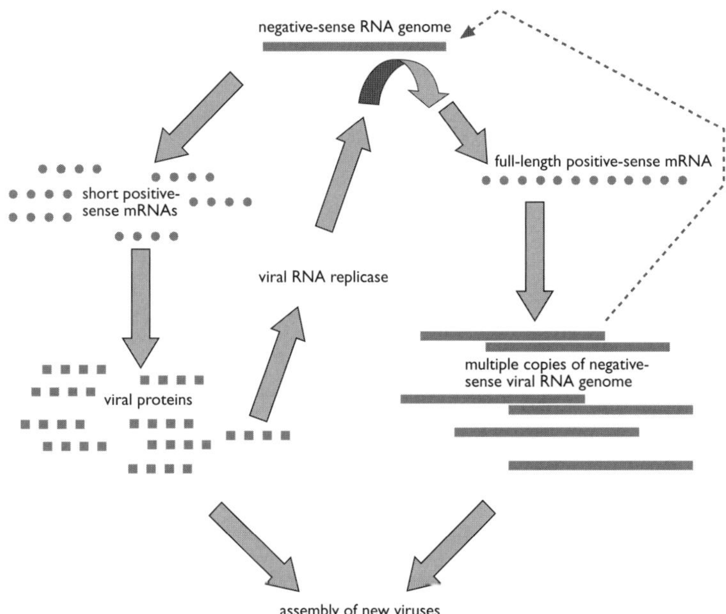

Fig 2.9 Replication of a 'negative-stranded' RNA virus
Source: Alastair J. Scott

We have mentioned the 'central dogma' which holds that information flows from DNA to RNA to protein. With the single-stranded RNA retroviruses, information can flow in the reverse direction, from RNA to DNA. When a retrovirus, such as HIV, infects a susceptible cell, a DNA copy of the viral RNA genes is made, forming an RNA–DNA double strand. The RNA strand disintegrates, and the DNA strand doubles up and physically integrates into the host cell DNA as a 'provirus'. The viral enzyme which catalyses these steps is reverse transcriptase (RT), discovered independently in 1970 by Howard Temin and David Baltimore, for which they were awarded a Nobel prize. The provirus can then be transcribed into viral RNA, using host RNA polymerase. Viruses are assembled and secreted from the host cells (Fig 2.10).

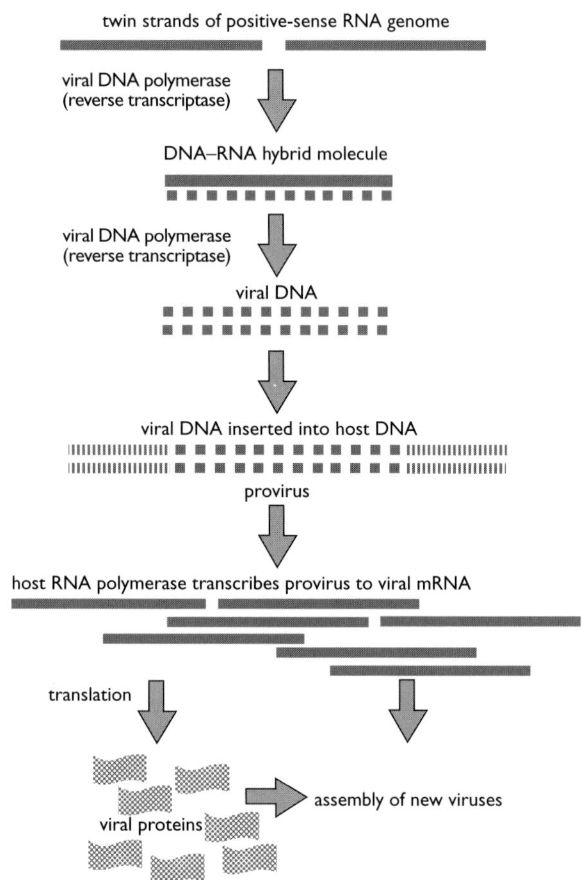

Fig 2.10 Replication of a retrovirus
Source: Alastair J. Scott

In contrast to bacteria, viruses replicate inefficiently. It has been estimated that less than 10% of the proteins and nucleic acid produced by viruses in the cell is assembled to form an infectious virus (Richman et al, 1984). This means that excess amounts of one or more virus components may accumulate in the host cell to form inclusion bodies. For example, in humans and most animals suffering from rabies, inclusions called Negri bodies can be seen by light microscopy in stained brain smears and are a definitive laboratory diagnostic test. While many virulent viruses can quickly shut down the host cell machinery, other viruses can adopt different strategies. For example, certain papillomaviruses can become intimately associated with the host DNA to the extent that the host cells become predisposed to becoming cancerous. The herpesviruses share the ability to remain latent in the host after initial infection, sometimes only producing disease years later. So viruses are not just cellular vandals, but agents capable of the most subtle interactions with their hosts. Indeed, this degree of molecular intimacy has led to speculation that viruses are pieces of DNA or RNA that have broken away from cellular nucleic acid and made successful bids for freedom (Tan and Niu, 1997). By now you may have a sense of viruses being 'apart' from other microbes; that viruses are on the *threshold* of life rather than being truly alive, and it might be interesting to explore this perception a little further.

Perhaps you have seen time-lapse films on television where a bacterium grows and divides into two, then four and so on. It is usually accompanied by some rather uninspired electronic music which trys to evoke a sense of mystery, and the screen fills with a heaving mass of microbes seemingly capable of multiplying indefinitely. What we see is well and truly alive. There is no doubt about it. If we give antibiotics to these bacteria, they gradually stop moving and die. It is uncomplicated. They were alive, and now they are dead. The music stops.

In contrast, when viruses are *outside* living cells, they are inert. They do not feed, they do not produce energy, they do not grow in size, they do not produce spores, they do not pass 'go' because they are not motile. However, when they are *inside* cells, viruses appear to be very much 'alive'. They can make vast numbers of new viruses, damage or kill the host cells, and produce disease. Alternatively, they may hide out in the host cell for a long time before eventually wreaking havoc. Clearly, many complex chemical reactions occur as a result of virus infection, but does this make the viruses themselves 'alive'?

An attempt to answer this might first involve dipping a toe into some philosophical waters to ask what is the meaning of life. One view says everything in the material world has a design or purpose behind it. This is *teleology*. However, according to Michael Young, a character in Stephen Fry's *Making History* (1996): 'The point is there *is* no point. That's the point.' So, a teleologist might say that viruses are alive and have a purpose, an aim, when they infect us. Indeed, 'viral strategy' is a commonly used term when replication is discussed. Michael Young, though, would have a more 'operational' view: it just happens – a molecular demolition derby in which the host comes off worst, sustaining great damage or dying. Viruses and cells: winners and losers. But is there not a more subtle relationship between viruses and cells? We have seen how cells and viruses use the same genetic code for making their component parts, how easily host enzymes can be adopted by viruses, and we can speculate that viruses may have originated from pieces of our own cellular material, evolved into the autonomous entities we know today, and are merely interacting with us. For example, some cancer-causing viruses carry 'cancer genes' which are altered genes they have acquired from host cells, and these genes can be transferred between cells. It is not inconceivable that viruses might even transfer genes that confer an evolutionary advantage. For instance, we could speculate that sperm or egg cells which have incorporated a 'beneficial' viral gene into their DNA could pass this advantage on to future generations. Although viruses are foreign agents in one sense, if they originated from cells in the first place, they could be regarded as merely coming back home. In the language of the shopping mall, 'viruses are us'.

As to whether viruses are alive or not, the answer is yes – and no; and it seems reasonable to say that examining the question probably enriches our understanding of this aspect of virology more than a simple yes or no answer might. In physics light is described as being particulate in nature, but it can also be described as having a wave-form. Perhaps we should think in a similar way about viruses. They can be simple disease-producing living organisms, or a complex collection of interacting chemicals which are more intimately involved in shaping our destinies than we might at first think.

References

Brooks, G. F., Butel, J. S., Ornston, L. N. (1991) General properties of viruses. In: *Jawetz, Melnick & Adelberg's Medical Microbiology*. East Norwalk, CT: Appleton & Lange, p. 380.

Fry, S. (1996) *Making History*. London: Hutchinson, p. 311.

Lehninger, A. L. (1972) *Biochemstry.* New York: Worth Publishers Inc., p. 5.

Richman, D. D., Cleveland, P. H., Redfield, D. C. et al (1984) Rapid viral diagnosis. *Journal of Infectious Diseases*; 149: 3, 298–310.

Smith, K. M. (1963) *Viruses*. Cambridge: Cambridge University Press, p. 45.

Tan, H., Niu, G. (1997) Endogenous origin of viruses. *Medical Hypotheses*; 49: 501–504.

3 Specimen collection

By a small sample we may judge of the whole piece.

Miguel de Cervantes (1547–1616), *Don Quixote*.

The financial exigencies of the National Health Service have required departments to undergo the rigours of medical audit, and laboratories are no exception. One aspect of this critical gaze includes a detailed scrutiny of specimens – and their accompanying request forms. Computerisation is an effective means of processing the data generated by laboratory tests, but to be properly efficient, certain minimum requirements need to be met. For example, it is an increasingly likely possibility that a badly filled-in request form will delay, or even disqualify, a specimen from being processed in the laboratory.

Badly completed request forms are easy to recognise, but it is impossible to distinguish between well- and badly-taken specimens. It is the responsibility of the clinician or nurse in charge to ensure that appropriate, well-taken specimens are collected, packaged, and transported to the laboratory, if meaningful results are expected in return. Large numbers of specimens are processed daily according to established protocols, so if urgent or exceptional tests are required, or an unusual problem arises, it is important to consult with the laboratory at an early stage to discuss individual cases.

The timing of specimen collection is especially important during the acute phase of virus infections. Virus shedding or viraemia is usually maximal before the onset of clinical illness, and often ceases by about five days from the onset of symptoms. By this time, the immune response against the virus is also getting under way so it is important to collect specimens as early in the disease as possible.

The choice of specimen is determined by the pathogenesis of the presumed disease. In diseases which are expressed on the skin or mucous membranes, specimens should be taken from the affected site. However, diseases of the central nervous system, non-vesicular rashes, congenital infections, and more generalised illnesses often require multiple sites to be sampled. The stability of viruses varies widely, with enveloped viruses generally more labile than non-enveloped viruses. For example, respiratory syncytial virus (RSV) is relatively fragile outside the body, compared to enteroviruses, which remain viable for many days in sewage or in water. Factors adversely affecting the stability of viruses are:

- drying
- heat
- freezing at around 0°C
- pH shock
- ultraviolet light
- oxidising agents

Specimens submitted for virus isolation are more likely to give positive results if the specimen:

- contains as much virus as possible at collection
- is in a suitable virus transport medium (VTM)
- is kept cold, but not frozen
- arrives in the laboratory promptly

Despite these strictures, some viruses can withstand prolonged storage and transport. A recent study (Coleman et al, 1998) that compared an overnight postal service with a more expensive same-day courier service found that virus isolation rates were similar. The five-month study period covered the winter months, the period of greatest respiratory viral activity, and most routine specimens submitted were included in the trial. It was concluded that viruses can be successfully isolated when specimens are transported overnight using a suitable VTM and first-class post.

Viruses can be transported in the specimen itself – for example, blood, urine, cerebrospinal fluid, nasopharyngeal secretions and faeces. When swabs are taken, the maximum amount of virus is on the swab at the time of collection, which is when the chances of successful isolation are greatest.

While some recommend bedside inoculation of cell-culture tubes, this is often impractical. So, to maintain viral infectivity during dispatch to the laboratory, the swab must be placed directly in a suitable VTM; dry swabs should not be sent. Herpes simplex virus has been shown to bind directly to calcium alginate, making it non-infectious, and for this reason calcium alginate swabs should not be used for the collection of virus specimens (Johnson, 1990). Specimen containers should be clearly labelled with the patient's name, date of birth, hospital and ward number, and the nature of the specimen.

VTM is usually available from diagnostic virus laboratories, typically in 3ml volumes in sterile bijoux bottles, and has a shelf-life of one month at 4°C. It typically consists of a balanced salt solution containing a buffering system to protect against pH changes, 10% protein to enhance virus stability, and antibiotics to prevent or minimise contamination by bacteria and fungi.

Specimens for virus isolation or detection should never be left at room temperature or in an incubator, but transported to the laboratory, on wet ice, without delay. While awaiting transport, specimens can be refrigerated at 4°C, with the virus remaining infectious for at least one or two days at this temperature. Do not freeze specimens; freeze-thawing is harmful to many viruses, and they rapidly loose infectivity.

UNIVERSAL, STANDARD AND ROUTINE BLOOD AND BODY SUBSTANCE PRECAUTIONS

Concerns over the risks of infection from the blood and body fluids of patients infected with the human immunodeficiency virus (HIV) led to the concept of 'universal blood and body fluid precautions', which were based on the principle that *all* patients should be assumed to be infectious for HIV and other blood-borne pathogens. In 1990 the UK Health Departments issued advice on Universal Precautions (UPs) which were to be applied when there was a risk of exposure to the blood or body fluids of *any* patient.

Originally, UPs applied to all body fluids, but were then modified to encompass only those fluids known to be associated with the spread of blood-borne viral pathogens, that is blood and blood-stained body fluids, amniotic, synovial, pleural, peritoneal, pericardial and cerebrospinal fluids, semen and vaginal secretions. However, it was accepted that pathogens found in other body substances, such as faeces, urine and sputum, represented major sources of infection. By applying UPs to the management of all body substances, the concept of Body Substance Isolation (BSI) sought to incorporate a policy for the prevention of blood-borne virus infections into an all-embracing one of prevention of nosocomial infection.

In 1996, the key elements of UPs and BSI were combined to give Standard Precautions, the basic features of which are shown in Table 3.1. Standard Precautions apply to blood, all body fluids, secretions and excretions except sweat, regardless of whether they contain visible blood, non-intact skin and mucous membranes (Kibbler, 1997).

Handwashing	After touching blood, body fluids, secretions, excretions and contaminated items, regardless of whether gloves are worn Immediately after removing gloves and between patients
Gloves	Wear when touching above fluids and items, mucous membranes and non-intact skin Remove after contact with material that may contain high content of micro-organisms and between patients
Masks and eyewear	Wear during procedures likely to generate splashes or sprays of above fluids
Gowns	Wear during procedures likely to generate splashes or sprays of the above fluids and likely to contaminate clothing
Equipment	Ensure appropriate cleaning of re-usable equipment between patients. Handle equipment soiled with the above fluids in a safe manner
Environmental control	Ensure adequate routine cleaning procedures
Linen	Handle soiled linen in a safe manner
Occupational health	Carefully dispose of all sharps. Do not recap needles. Take care when handling all sharp instruments
Patient placement	Place a patient who contaminates the environment or who does not (or cannot be expected to) assist in maintaining appropriate hygiene or environmental control in a private room

Table 3.1 Outline of Standard Precautions

Source: Reprinted from C. C. Kibbler (1997), with permission of CAB International, Wallingford, Oxon., OX10 8DE

Specimens for virus diagnosis

The Infection Control Team in each hospital will have an Infection Control Policy Manual which contains protocols describing the correct procedures for the safe collection of specimens for pathological examination. These must be followed. Below are some additional comments relating to specimens for virological examination.

Blood

The standard serological diagnosis of virus infections has long been based on the examination of appropriately timed clotted blood samples (5–10 ml), which yield adequate serum for multiple tests. The blood samples can be refrigerated overnight, or over a weekend, without affecting their usefulness in tests. The range of tests for which blood samples are required has recently widened.

The increasing use of molecular techniques such as the polymerase chain reaction (PCR) has revolutionised diagnostic virology by providing powerful tools for the detection and measurement of the amount of virus, or 'viral load' to be made. For example, many individuals infected with HIV are routinely monitored for HIV viral load to assess their response to antiviral therapy, and there is evidence that a high cytomegalovirus (CMV) load is associated with an increased risk of progression to CMV disease, especially in solid-organ transplant recipients and in HIV-infected individuals (Boeckh and Boivin, 1998).

As a result, there is now a wider range of more stringent blood-collection schedules for virology than before. For example: blood tubes with or without anticoagulant may be required in specific circumstances; there is often a need for minimum volumes of blood to be drawn if subsequent results are to be meaningful; the timing between blood collection and laboratory processing is critical for some tests; and the storage conditions of blood samples prior to processing may vary.

Taking blood is a high-risk, exposure-prone procedure, with accidental blood exposure during phlebotomy the main cause of occupationally acquired HIV infection (Bouvet, 1997). The blood-borne viruses of most concern to nurses are HIV, and those of hepatitis B (for which there is an effective vaccine), hepatitis C and hepatitis D; the small risk of acquiring CMV should be borne in mind by those nurses in the child-bearing age group. Needlestick injuries account for about 80% of all accidental exposures to blood, with most occurring after blood has been taken (Griffiths, 1997).

It is possible to reduce the risks of acquiring blood-borne infections by using safe blood-collection devices (Fig 3.1), adopting safe practices (Table 3.2), and avoiding hazardous practices (Fig 3.2).

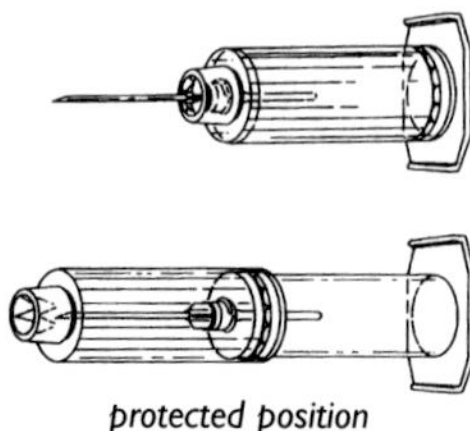

VACUTAINER® Brand Safety-Lok™
■ Becton Dickinson
Single use vacuum tube/needle holder with protective sliding sleeve that pushes forward after use and locks in place

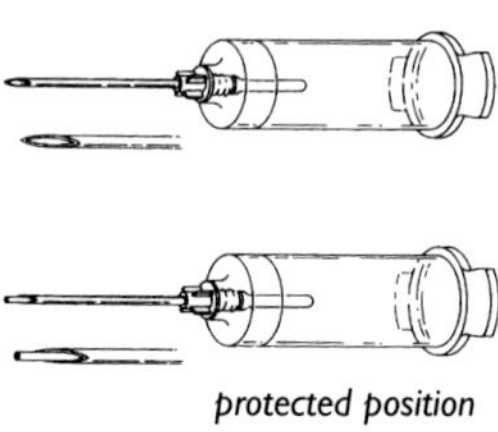

Punctur-Guard™ ■ Bio-Plexus
After final tube of blood is drawn, blunt internal needle is activated by forward pressure of vacuum tube. Needle point is blunted before it is removed from patient

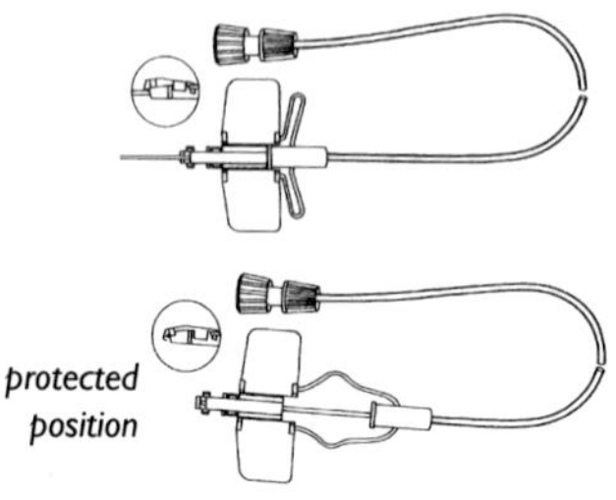

Angel Wing™ Safety Needle
■ Sherwood Medical
Stainless steel barrier tip is advanced forward to end of needle, locking over point as needle is withdrawn from patient; one-handed activation

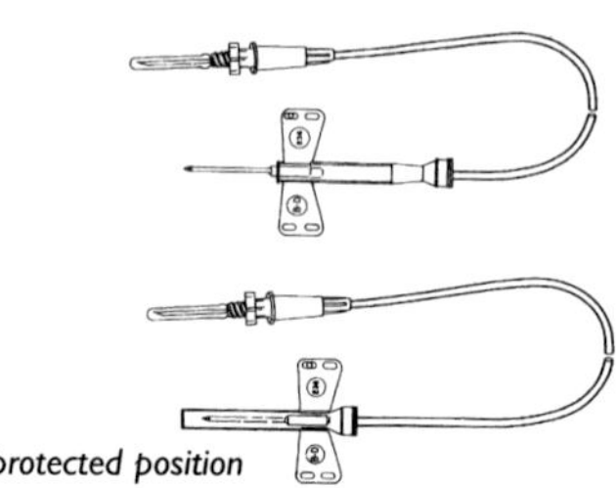

VACUTAINER® Brand Safety-Lok™
Winged Needle ■ Becton Dickinson
After removal from patient, safety shield is advanced forward and locks in place beyond needle tip

Fig 3.1 Safety products related to blood drawing

Source: Reprinted from J. Jagger and M. Bentley (1997), with permission of CAB International, Wallingford, Oxon., OX10 8DE

Fig 3.1 continued

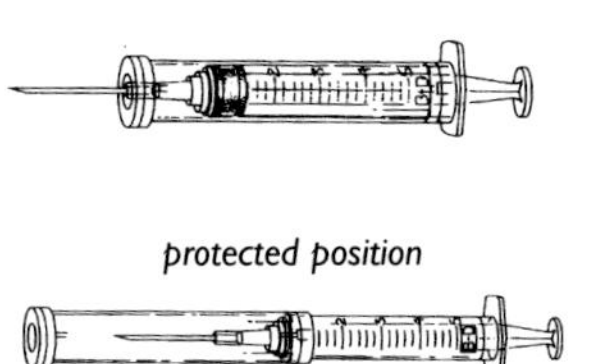

B-D Safety-Lock™ ■ Becton Dickinson
Needle guard has protective sliding sleeve that pushes forward after use and locks in place. Note: the 10cc syringe with the shield locked in place can accept a 3cc to 10cc vacuum tube, allowing injection of blood into tube with shielded needle

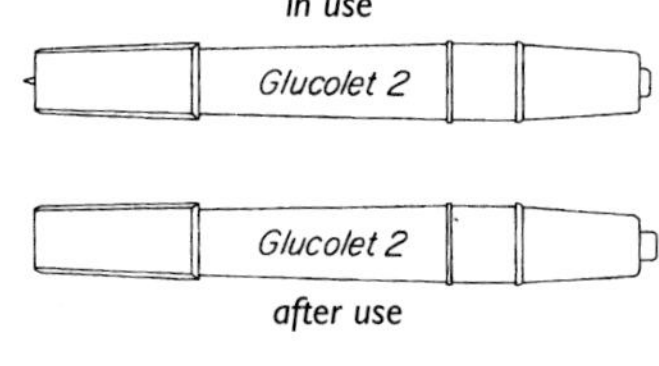

Glucolet 2™ Retracting Lancet ■ Miles, Inc./Diagnostic Division
Disposable lancet is fitted to reusable spring-loaded holder. When activated, lancet instantly protracts and retracts; retracted lancet is removed from holder for disposal

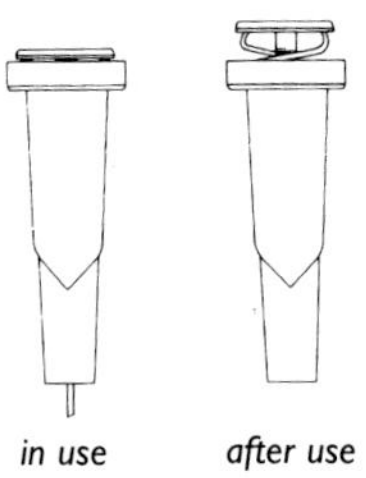

MICROTAINER™ Brand Safety Flow Lancet ■ Becton Dickinson
Self-contained lancet is manually activated and automatically retracts when activating lever is released

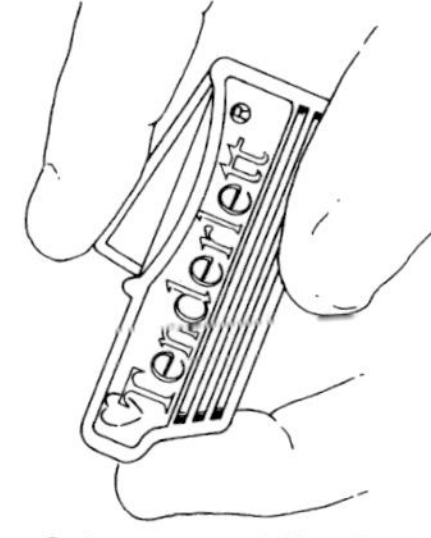

Tenderlet ® Automated Skin Incision Device ■ International Technidyne Corporation
When device is triggered, surgical steel blade swiftly protracts and then automatically retracts. Design precludes inadvertent reuse

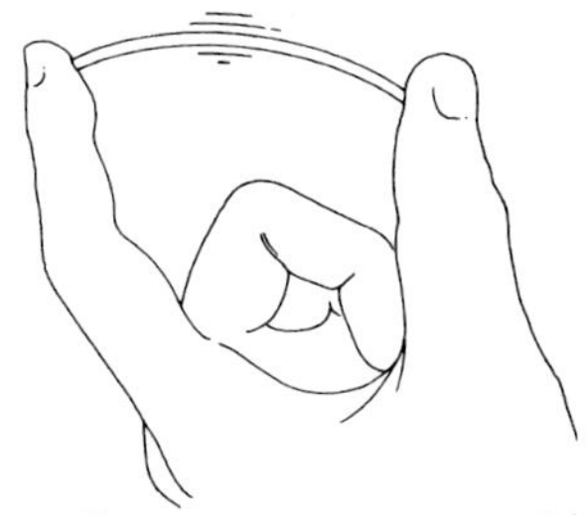

SafeCrit™ Plastic Microhematocrit Tube ■ Norfolk Scientific
Capillary tube made of plastic avoids hazard of glass breakage

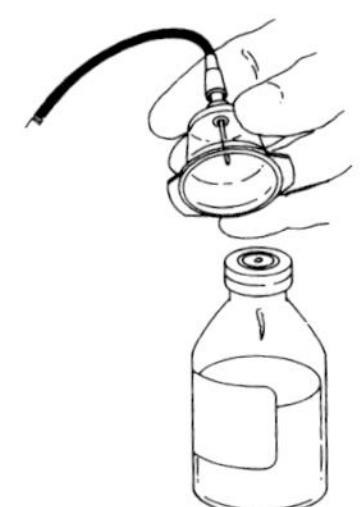

BACTEC ® Direct Draw Adapter ■ Becton Dickinson. Designed for blood culture procedures. Vacuum vial and covered needle safety adaptor allow blood to be drawn directly into culture medium, avoiding need to inject into specimen container

Fig 3.1 continued

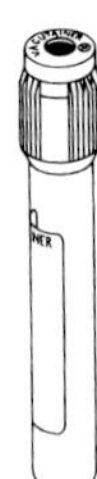

HEMOGARD VACUTAINER® Brand Vacuum Tube Stopper ■ Becton Dickinson
Rigid stopper grips outside of tube; intended to reduce risk of tube breakage and blood splash when removing stoppers

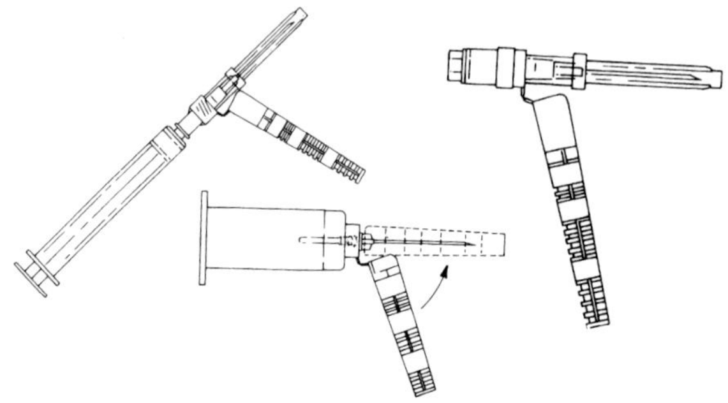

Needle-ProT™ Needle Protection Devices ■ SIMS: Smiths Industries Medical Systems
Hinged sheath engages over needle; used needle is pressed into Needle-Pro device using one hand. Comes in three configurations. (1) Needle-Pro: Basic needle protection device; can be used for arterial blood drawing. (2) Cartridge Needle-Pro: Combines hypodermic needle cartridge with Needle-Pro sheath. (3) Venipuncture Needle-Pro: Disposable blood collection tube holder and integral needle protection device

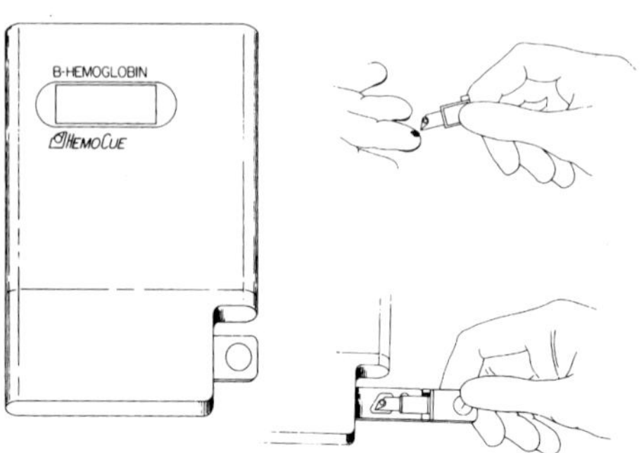

HemoCue® Hematocrit Reader ■ HemoCue, Inc.
Uses flat plastic cuvette to contain blood sample for hematocrit determination. Cuvette is inserted directly into reader, avoiding need for centrifugation

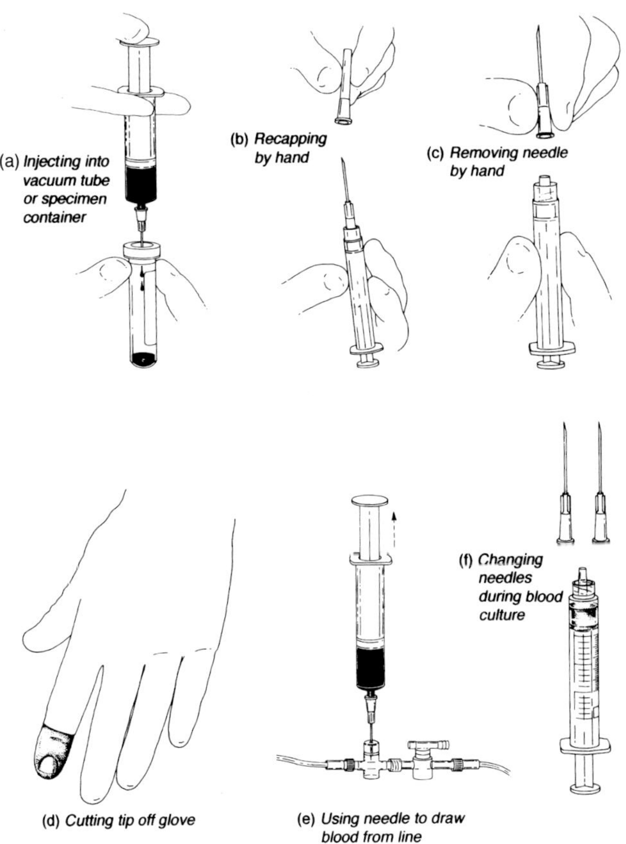

Fig 3.2 Six hazardous practices to avoid

Source: Reprinted from J. Jagger and M. Bentley (1997), with permission of CAB International, Wallingford, Oxon., OX10 8DE

- Avoid or reduce use of sharps wherever possible

  If unavoidable take extreme care in handling and disposal
- Do not re-sheathe needles wherever possible
  If unavoidable use a re-sheathing device or one hand only
- Use good basic hygiene practice, especially adequate handwashing
  Avoid hand to mouth/eye contact
- Protect breaks in skin with waterproof adhesive dressings and disposable gloves
- Ensure safe disposal of all clinical waste and sharps by incineration
  Where incineration is not available on site ensure safe handling and transport to incinerator

Where blood or body fluid splashes are likely

- Wear waterproof or water-resistant protective clothing
  Protect eyes with goggles, mouth with mask or visor
- Ensure safe decontamination of equipment and hard surfaces

Precautions in use of equipment in operating theatre, labour ward, etc.

- In lengthy procedures routine change of gloves is necessary in addition to when they are punctured
- Place prepared needles and needleholder with points down to prevent snagging of gloves
- Use magnetic pad or emesis bowl to avoid placing instruments directly into hands or, at least, ensure visual contact when passing instruments
  Use thimble to protect index finger of non-dominant hand
  Use knife blade holder for mechanical removal of blade with one hand
- Use alternatives to sutures, e.g. 'superglue'

Table 3.2 Reducing the risks of acquiring blood-borne infections
Source: Reprinted from G. Griffiths (1997), with permission of CAB International, Wallingford, Oxon., OX10 8DE

Nose and throat swabs

Well-taken throat swabs should sample both sides of the tonsillar area, and the posterior wall of the pharynx (Somerville, 1983). Nose and throat swabs should be broken off into the same bottle of VTM and gently shaken.

Nasopharyngeal aspirate (NPA)

These specimens are commonly submitted from paediatric patients in whom evidence of respiratory virus infection is sought. A well-taken NPA specimen provides more cells for the detection and isolation of common respiratory viruses than a nose and throat swab.

Sputum

Although viruses can be identified in and isolated from sputum specimens, they may have originated in the oropharynx. Sputum is often toxic to cell cultures, and many diagnostic virology laboratories discourage this specimen from being sent. However, laboratories testing for *Pneumocystis carinii* pneumonia (PCP) will accept induced sputum samples.

Bronchoalveolar lavage

This specimen is preferable to sputum and is increasingly used, particularly in the evaluation of the immunocompromised, especially adults. For example, it has been shown (Englund et al, 1996) that a bronchoalveolar lavage (BAL) specimen is more sensitive than a nasal-wash/throat-swab specimen for the rapid diagnosis of RSV disease in immunocompromised adults. In addition, BAL is the specimen of choice for PCP testing.

Cerebrospinal fluid (CSF)

This should be collected in a sterile, plastic Universal container. At least one ml of CSF is preferred; the specimen may be cultured and/or used for antibody and molecular tests, and some may be needed for posting to specialist reference laboratories. However, we may soon anticipate PCR techniques which require only small volumes of CSF. Bloody samples may contain antibodies which could inhibit any virus present; 'clean' CSF is preferred.

Urine and faeces

These specimens should be put into sterile, plastic Universal containers. While good-sized specimens are preferred by the laboratory, there is no need for Universal containers to be filled to the brim with urine, nor completely packed with faeces.

Vomitus

This is an inappropriate specimen for virology, and should not be sent.

Vesicle fluid

The fluid of several vesicles should be aspirated into a 1ml tuberculin syringe fitted with a 25-gauge needle. The needle is then transferred to a Universal container. Vesicle fluid allows electron microscopy to be performed on an undiluted specimen. The needle can then be flushed out with a small amount of VTM, which can be tested by immunofluorescence and/or cultured. If vesicle fluid cannot be obtained, a swab of the base of a freshly opened vesicle is the next best thing; this is broken into a bottle of VTM and agitated gently. Vesicle crusts should not be sent; they are unlikely to contain viable virus.

References

Boeckh, M., Boivin, G. (1998) Quantitation of cytomegalovirus: methodologic aspects and clinical applications. *Clinical Microbiology Reviews*; 11: 3, 533–554.

Bouvet, E. (1997) Phlebotomy. In: Collins, C. H., Kennedy, D. A. (eds) *Occupational Blood-borne Infections: Risk and Management*. Wallingford: CAB International.

Coleman, T. J., Clark, G., Caul, E. O. et al (1998) How well do viruses survive during transport? *Communicable Disease and Public Health*; 1: 2, 127–129.

Englund, J. A., Piedra, P. A., Jewell A. et al (1996) Rapid diagnosis of respiratory syncytial virus infections in immunocompromised adults. *Journal of Clinical Microbiology*; 34: 7, 1649–1653.

Griffiths, G. (1997) Nursing care. In: Collins, C. H., Kennedy, D. A. (eds) *Occupational Blood-borne Infections: Risk and Management*. Wallingford: CAB International.

Jagger, J., Bentley, M. (1997) Percutaneous blood exposure data: 58 hospitals in the USA. In: Collins, C. H., Kennedy, D. A. (eds) *Occupational Blood-borne Infections: Risk and Management*. Wallingford: CAB International.

Johnson, F. B. (1990) Transport of viral specimens. *Clinical Microbiology Reviews*; 3: 2, 120–131.

Kibbler, C. C. (1997) Universal Precautions and the advent of Standard Precautions: a review. In: Collins, C. H., Kennedy, D. A. (eds) *Occupational Blood-borne Infections: Risk and Management*. Wallingford: CAB International.

Somerville, R. G. (1983) Specimens for virus diagnosis. In: Somerville, R. G. *Essential Clinical Virology*. Oxford: Blackwell Scientific Publications.

4 Laboratory diagnosis

The diagnosis of disease is often easy, often difficult, and often impossible.

Peter Mere Latham (1789–1875).

The traditional complaint that by the time a virology laboratory has made a diagnosis, the patient has either died or gone home is an increasingly untenable point of view. The availability of rapid diagnostic techniques means that results can often be obtained within a few hours of receipt of specimens. The trend towards rapid diagnosis has been driven by several factors. The availability of effective antiviral therapy and its appropriate application require timely, specific laboratory diagnoses. For example, the ability to distinguish between herpes simplex and varicella zoster in an immunocompromised patient can help to determine the choice of a particular therapeutic regime. Transplantation is an increasingly preferred option in the treatment of organ dysfunctions and some malignancies. However, infection is the main cause of death in transplant recipients, and an efficient laboratory service providing quick results is needed through all stages of the transplantation process. Rapid and accurate diagnosis is also required for the effective control of nosocomial infections in hospitals, to study outbreaks of viral disease in the community, and to investigate suspected virus infections during pregnancy.

The virus laboratory is not just geared to achieving rapid test results. Screening tests provide information on the immune status of patients in relation to different viruses. For example, antenatal screening identifies those women at risk from rubella virus infection, and screening sera for antibody to hepatitis B virus helps to monitor the efficacy of hepatitis B immunisation among vaccinees. Additionally, the virus laboratory has a role in ruling out the involvement of particular viruses prior to or during a course of treatment: for example, in screening the serum of prospective transplant recipients/donors for evidence of the viruses of hepatitis B, hepatitis C, human immunodeficiency virus (HIV), herpes simplex (HSV), varicella zoster (VZV) and cytomegalovirus (CMV).

Most virus laboratories provide an on-call service to process urgent specimens, and consultant scientific and medical staff are available to advise users on whether an 'urgent' specimen is truly urgent, and how generally to make the most efficient and cost-effective use of the service. This is increasingly important as economic constraints mean that the rationale for doing certain tests is now subject to greater scrutiny than before.

Laboratory diagnosis is based on:

- growing viruses in cells and observing their effect on the cells
- the direct detection of viruses or their antigenic or nucleic acid components
- serology (the detection of antibodies to specific viral proteins)

Cell culture

The isolation of viruses in cell culture has been a cornerstone of diagnostic virology for over 50 years. Most virus laboratories have a dedicated cell-culture section supplying test-tubes with a single layer of cells, growing on part of the inner surface, bathed in one ml of nutrient medium. The tubes are incubated at 37°C on their sides in large, slowly rotating drums. When specimens are received, they are either inoculated directly into cell cultures or pre-treated. If, for example, genital or throat or eye swabs are received in virus transport medium (VTM), they are agitated to dislodge virus-containing cells from the swab into the medium, and then about 0.2ml of the specimen is added to appropriate tubes. With stool specimens, an approximate 10% suspension is made in 10ml of a balanced salt solution containing antibiotics and sterile glass beads. After agitation, the suspension is spun hard in a centrifuge, and 0.2ml of the supernatant (the clear liquid obtained) is inoculated. Cloudy urines or bloody cerebrospinal fluids (CSFs) can be clarified by gentle centrifugation before inoculation. Respiratory specimens are incubated at 33°C, as this temperature approximates more to that of the respiratory tract, and the rest at 36–37°C. Thereafter, tubes are examined, using a light microscope, two or three times a week for evidence of virus growth.

Many viruses, when added to susceptible cell-cultures, will produce characteristic degenerative changes in the cells which can be observed microscopically. These are called cytopathic effects (CPE); *pathic*, 'producing disease in'; *cyto*, 'cells'. A larger diagnostic laboratory might typically use three cell lines; cells derived from monkey kidney tissue, human embryonic lung or human foreskin fibroblasts, and transformed human epithelial cells. Different cell lines have different susceptibilities to different viruses. For example, the viruses of influenza and mumps are most readily detected in monkey kidney, HSV grows in all three cell lines, whereas CMV will produce a CPE only in fibroblasts (Fig 4.1). The isolation of a virus in cell culture does not *necessarily* mean that it has caused the disease under investigation. For example, poliovirus vaccine might be isolated from the faeces of a recently vaccinated infant suffering from a common cold, whose respiratory specimen has yielded a rhinovirus.

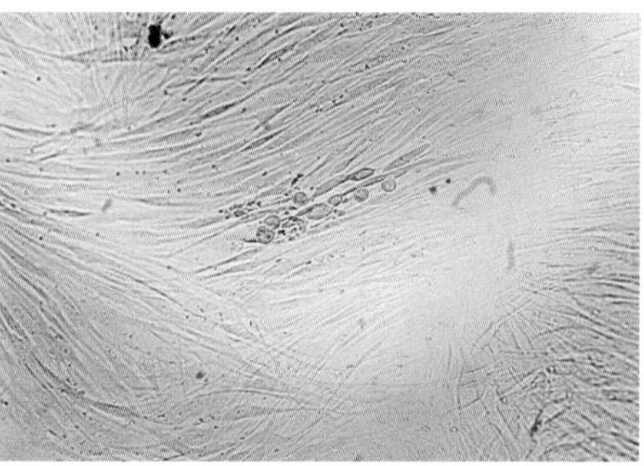

Fig 4.1 The cytopathic effect of cytomegalovirus seen in human embryo fibroblast cells
Source: Courtesy of Mr A. J. MacAulay, Regional Clinical Virology Laboratory, City Hospital, Edinburgh EH10 5SB

In theory a single infectious virus can produce a CPE, making virus isolation very sensitive. In addition, using more than one cell line allows the detection of multiple viruses in a specimen. For example, a throat swab might yield influenzavirus in monkey kidney, and HSV in fibroblasts and human epithelial cells. However, virus isolation has two main limitations. First, some viruses may take a long time to grow, so, for example, whereas enteroviruses might produce a CPE after overnight incubation, CMV can take a month. Attempts to address this problem have been made by applying chemical and physical methods which enhance the early detection of some viruses. In shell vial cultures, cells are grown on round coverslips in small vials instead of culture tubes. When a specimen is added, the vial is spun at high speed, allowing the rapid entry of virus into the cell. The vial is incubated for one to two days, and then tested for the presence of a particular virus by immunofluorescence, described below. The second limitation of conventional culture is that many viruses cannot be easily isolated in the cell cultures available to routine diagnostic laboratories. These include rotaviruses, Epstein-Barr virus (EBV), human papilloma viruses, hepatitis A, B, C, D and E viruses, and HIV. Other techniques, such as direct detection and serology, are required.

Direct detection

This refers to the direct detection of a virus or a viral component by microscopy, immunological detection or nucleic acid detection.

Some viruses may produce virus-specific structures within cells called inclusion bodies which, when stained, can be seen with a light microscope, and are a useful diagnostic aid. Inclusion bodies can be in the nucleus (for example, HSV), the cytoplasm (for example Negri bodies of rabies) or both (for example, measles).

While the light microscope can reach magnifications of around ×1,200, the electron microscope can magnify up to about ×300,000, enabling virus structure to be distinguished. The electron microscope (Fig 4.2) has been particularly successful in the examination of faeces specimens from patients with diarrhoea and vomiting (DV). Many of the agents responsible for gastroenteritis and DV cannot be easily grown, and electron microscopy (EM) is a favoured diagnostic method for detecting human caliciviruses, astroviruses and small round-structured viruses: it is simple and quick, with results possible within minutes of receipt of a specimen. Similarly, poxviruses such as molluscum contagiosum and orf, which have distinctive shapes, can be usefully diagnosed by EM. However, EM is expensive, requires a skilled operator, and only larger reference laboratories are likely to have an EM facility. Another disadvantage is in sensitivity, with at least 10^6 viruses per ml required for a positive result. In addition, viruses in the same family cannot be distinguished from each other. For example, a vesicle fluid specimen containing herpesvirus could be HSV (herpes simplex virus) or VZV (varicella zoster virus). EM is a tool best used selectively and to augment other diagnostic tests when appropriate.

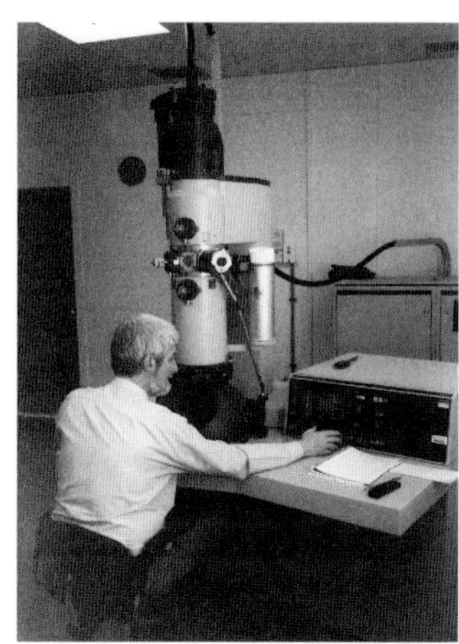

Fig 4.2 An electron microscope
Source: Courtesy of Mr D. Notman, Dept of Medical Microbiology, University of Edinburgh, Edinburgh EH8 9AG

The immunological detection of viruses, or their components, is based on the antigen-antibody reaction. An antigen is usually a protein which, when introduced into an animal, induces the production of circulating antibodies which can react with the antigen. Immunofluorescence staining is widely used in many laboratories for the rapid detection of viral antigens in specimens. Fluorescein isothiocyanate (FITC) is a green dye which can be chemically attached, or conjugated, to an antibody without interfering with its ability to react with an antigen when it meets one. The commercial availability, in kit form, of highly specific monoclonal antibodies to a wide range of viruses helps to ensure that results of high quality are obtained with these robust and reliable tests.

This is how it works. Suppose it is winter time with respiratory syncytial virus (RSV) rampant in the community. Nasopharyngeal secretions are taken from an infant with bronchiolitis and sent to the laboratory. After processing to remove mucus and bits of breakfast, nasal epithelial cells are transferred to a clean glass slide, air-dried, and dipped in acetone for 10 minutes to 'fix' the cells to the glass. Next, a drop of RSV antibody conjugated to FITC is placed over the cells and the slide is incubated at 37°C for 15 minutes. If RSV antigens are present in the cells, they will react with the conjugated antibody and form a firm bond. After incubation, the slide is rinsed, dried, mounted with a coverslip, and read using a microscope equipped to detect fluorescent light (Fig 4.3). Positive samples will show one or more cells with bright apple-green areas of fluorescence in their cytoplasm (Fig 4.4). In negative samples such specific fluorescence is absent. Commercial reagents are routinely available to detect viral antigens such as influenzavirus types A and B, parainfluenza virus types

1, 2 and 3, adenovirus, HSV types 1 and 2, and VZV. This direct procedure can also be applied to cell-culture tubes showing a CPE; in this case, some cells are scraped off the glass, placed on a slide, dried, fixed, and then tested with a conjugated antibody to the presumed virus. Properly fixed specimens are stable. This means that small laboratories, for example at hospitals without their own virology centre, can prepare and fix specimens onto slides and post them to a reference virus laboratory for appropriate testing.

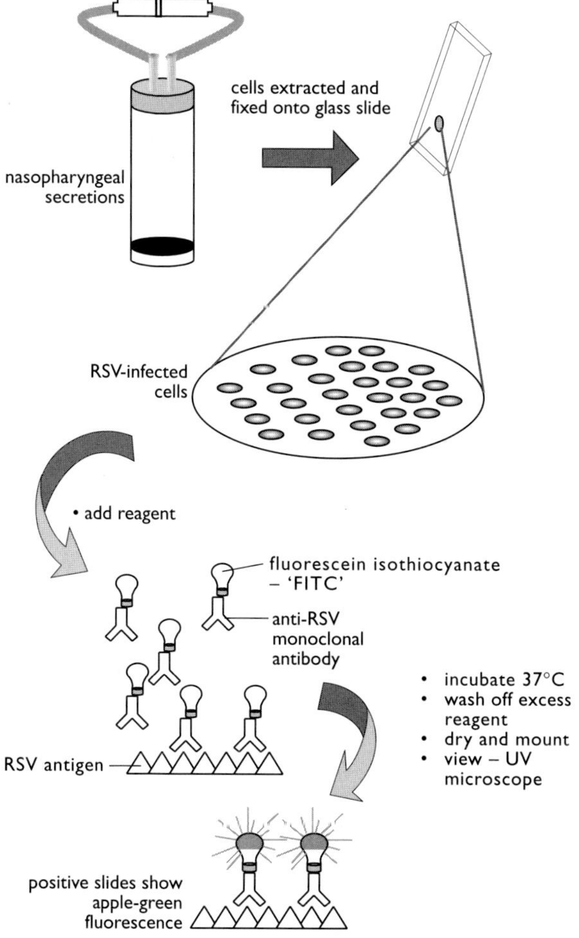

Fig 4.3 Direct immunofluorescence
Source: Alistair J. Scott

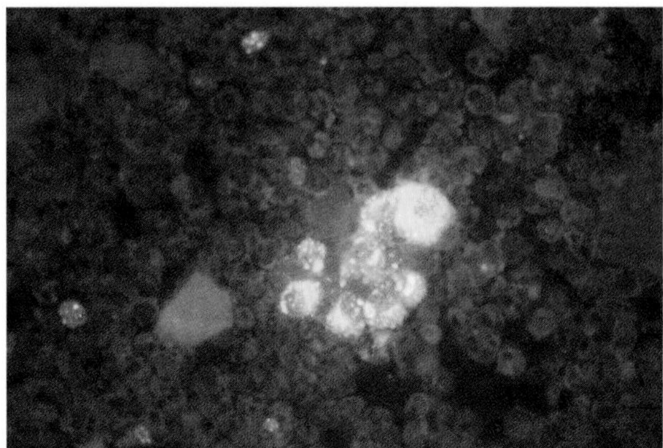

Fig 4.4 RSV-infected nasopharyngeal cells detected by direct immunofluorescence. Magnification x400
Source: Regional Clinical Virology Laboratory, City Hospital, Edinburgh EH10 5SB

With immunofluorescence, the 'indicator' is FITC attached to the antibody. In the enzyme immunoassay (EIA), an enzyme, such as horseradish peroxidase, is attached to the antibody. When a suitable substrate is added, the enzyme initiates a chemical reaction resulting in a colour change that can be read photometrically by machine, or observed microscopically or with the naked eye. Immunofluorescence and EIA share the same biological principle of an antigen-antibody reaction; only the indicator system differs.

In 1993 Kary Mullis, the inventor of the polymerase chain reaction (PCR), was awarded a Nobel prize for medicine. The PCR has become a powerful tool for the analysis of nucleic acids, and has seen many applications in all branches of biology. In diagnostic virology it is the fastest-growing of the direct-detection methods for many viruses which cannot be easily isolated by conventional cell culture.

We have seen how the genetic information of nucleic acids is contained in the sequence of bases which determines the proteins which are produced. Virus nucleic acids have unique base sequences, and for many viruses the complete base sequence has been determined. This makes PCR directly applicable to virus diagnosis. Let us take HIV as an example. A blood sample is treated to extract some host deoxyribonucleic acid (DNA), into which HIV has integrated in the form of DNA. There are three main elements to PCR. First, the DNA is heated to about 94°C to separate the two strands. Next, bases which are complementary to a particular HIV sequence are added, and the mixture cooled down to 42°C. Finally, using a polymerase enzyme at 72°C, these 'primer' bases are then extended along the length of the HIV segment which is sought. When the extension is complete, the whole three-stage cycle is repeated. With each cycle, the number of HIV sequences doubles. After a typical PCR of around 30 cycles, millions of copies could be made. These copies can be detected by transferring them to gels and staining them to show up the presence of HIV nucleic acid. PCR is so sensitive that one infected blood mononuclear cell in a million can sometimes be detected. Although a few commercially produced PCRs are available in kit form, they are very expensive and many laboratories have developed their own 'in-house' PCRs. Quality control is a major consideration in PCR work, and each phase of the process requires a separate room where stringent precautions to prevent contamination of the reactants must be undertaken. In spite of these potential drawbacks, PCR is likely to become a 'gold standard' against which other direct-detection methods are judged.

Serology

Although the PCR has focused attention on direct methods, the detection of virus-specific antibody is of great importance in the diagnosis of acute infections, in determining the immune status of individuals, and in the collection of epidemiological information. Indeed, the use of automated technology which can be easily integrated with new, sophisticated, rapid serological assays means that diagnostic serology will continue to be a powerful tool.

In humans, antibodies are proteins called immunoglobulins, of which there are five types; immunoglobulin G (IgG), IgM, IgA, IgD and IgE. IgG and IgM are the most keenly sought antibodies in serological diagnosis. When the immune system is first exposed to a virus, IgM antibodies are the first to appear, and usually reach peak levels after about a fortnight, before declining after two to three months to an undetectable concentration. The presence of IgM usually indicates a current or recent infection. In contrast, IgG antibodies reach their peak concentrations after about a month, but remain elevated for many years or for life. When a reinfection with the same or a similar virus occurs, the IgM response may be very low or undetectable, whereas high concentrations of IgG antibodies are rapidly produced, and will provide long-term protection.

Little is known of the precise roles played by IgD and IgE in the immune response to a virus, and these antibodies can, at present, be ignored in terms of laboratory diagnosis. More is known about the role of IgA in virus infections. As well as being found in the serum, IgA can be found in secretions. A relatively high concentration of this secretory IgA is produced in response to viruses that multiply in the mucosa of the respiratory, gastrointestinal and urogenital tracts, and is the first line of defence against local virus infections. However, in general, the IgA response is too inconsistent to find widespread application in routine testing for virus-specific IgA.

Antibodies are most often sought in serum specimens. However, saliva and urine are two specimens in which antibodies can be detected, and the advantages of such non-invasive specimens in virological diagnosis have been reported (Mortimer and Parry, 1991). For example, they are painless, non-invasive and simple to collect; their collection is less hazardous to subject and investigator alike, and they are better suited to investigations of large outbreaks, and for high-risk groups.

The three 'traditional' methods of detecting virus-specific antibodies are complement fixation, haemagglutination inhibition and neutralisation tests. However, newer, more sensitive immunometric assays, such as EIAs

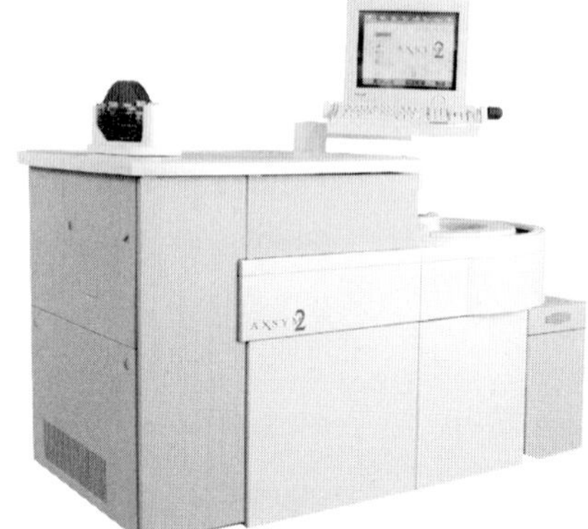

Fig 4.5 An automated laboratory analyser
Source: Courtesy of Abbott Diagnostics, Maidenhead, Berkshire SL6 4XL

are increasingly replacing these older methods, especially in busy reference laboratories. We have seen how EIAs can be used to directly detect an 'unknown' antigen in a specimen. In diagnostic serology EIAs use known antigens to determine whether specific antibodies are present in the patient's serum. The availability of automated assay systems (Fig 4.5), or analysers, based on microparticle EIA technology (Fig 4.6) permits the rapid testing of small numbers or, alternatively, large batches of sera. Let us consider an example.

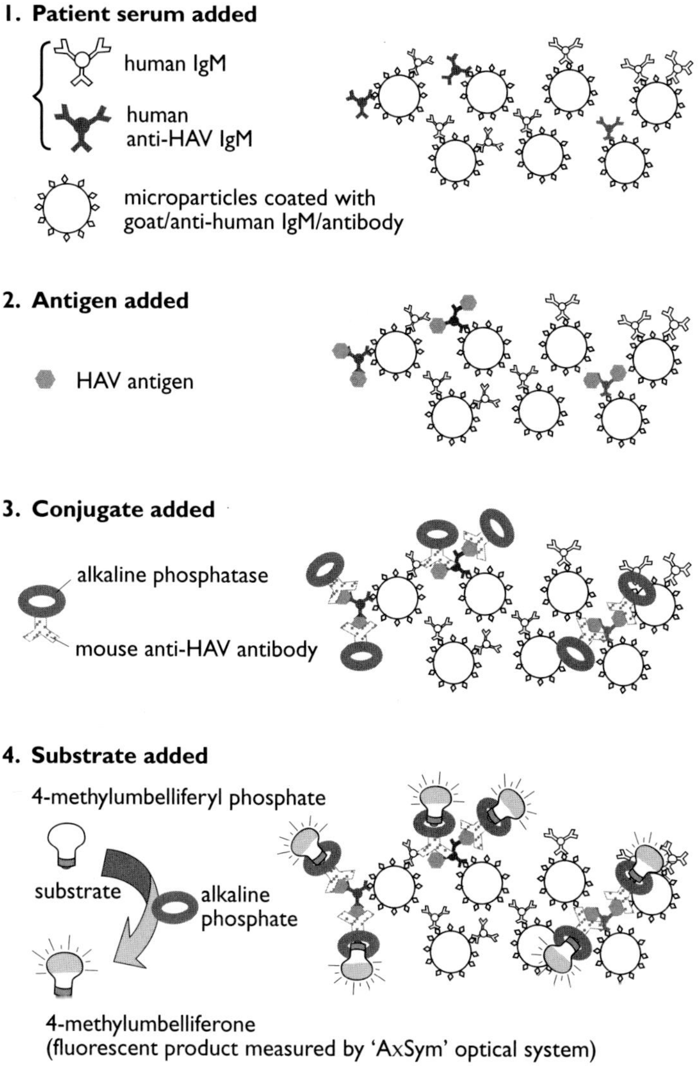

Fig 4.6 Microparticle EIA technology
Source: Alastair J. Scott

A patient with hepatitis A may be clinically indistinguishable from one with hepatitis B, necessitating a laboratory diagnosis. In an acute case of hepatitis A infection, hepatitis A-specific IgM antibody will appear in the patient's serum. To test for hepatitis A IgM, the patient's serum is added to microparticles coated with anti-human antibody. IgM in the serum binds to the microparticles. Hepatitis A antigen is added. If hepatitis A-specific IgM is in the patient's serum, hepatitis A antigen will bind to it on the microparticle. Next, an anti-hepatitis A antibody, with an enzyme tagged on, is added. This will bind to the hepatitis A antigen on the microparticle. Lastly, a substrate for the enzyme to act on is added. This produces a fluorescent colour change that is detected and measured by an optical system in the analyser. The convenience of such systems is that the operator only has to add the serum and read the result minutes later; all other stages are done by the machine.

As NHS trusts currently favour a multidisciplinary approach as one means of attaining greater efficiency and cost savings, it is likely that automated, user-friendly analysers will become increasingly used in the future. Thus HIV serology might be done side-by-side with syphilis serology, for example, blurring the traditional separation that has existed between virology and bacteriology. From a nursing perspective, as near-patient testing becomes more widespread, it seems possible that nursing staff in the not too distant future, might be involved in a wider range of ward-side, if not bedside tests than is currently seen. This will demand more collaboration between the ward and the laboratory, and raises the question of the role of laboratory diagnosis in nurses' training.

REFERENCES

Mortimer, P. P., Parry, J. V. (1991) Non-invasive diagnosis: are saliva and urine specimens adequate substitutes for blood? *Reviews in Medical Virology*; 1: 73–78.

5 The respiratory tract

And in this harsh world draw thy breath in pain,
To tell my story.

William Shakespeare (1564–1616), *Hamlet*.

Along with smoke, pollen, soot and dust, we breathe in an estimated 10,000 microbes each day (Mims, 1987). With such a daily challenge to its integrity, the hairs, mucus, cilia and macrophages of the respiratory tract together contrive to minimise the numbers of uninvited guests *en pension* in the airways.

Those particles making it through the coarse filtering follicular forests of each nostril will find themselves borne to the back of the throat on the 'mucociliary escalator' and swallowed. This escalator consists of ciliated epithelial cells lining the nasal cavity and most of the lower respiratory tract, which are daily charged with an estimated 10–100 ml of mucus from those sites. Small particles trapped in the mucus are gently, but firmly wafted up the respiratory tract, away from the lungs, to be swallowed; smaller particles managing to reach the alveoli will have escaped the mucociliary escalator only to encounter alveolar macrophages eager to phagocytose and digest the invaders.

Despite such barriers to infection, most acute infectious diseases worldwide are acquired through the respiratory or gastrointestinal tracts, with acute viral respiratory infections the commonest infections in developed countries. While droplet spread is a significant means of transmission, the hands play an equally important role. Most acute viral respiratory illnesses are caused by influenzaviruses, parainfluenza viruses, respiratory syncytial virus (RSV), rhinoviruses, adenoviruses and coronaviruses. Other viruses can cause acute respiratory illness, but are better known for other disease manifestations; these include measles virus, herpes simplex virus, enteroviruses and Epstein-Barr virus. Adenoviruses and rhinoviruses can cause illness throughout the year, whereas RSV, influenzaviruses and parainfluenza viruses have seasonal activity (Figs 5.1–5.3).

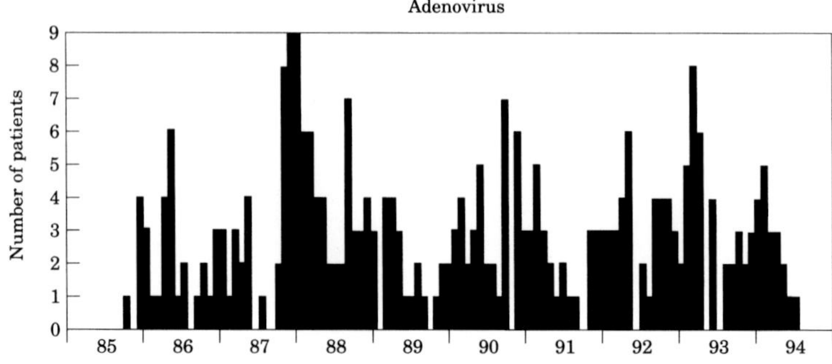

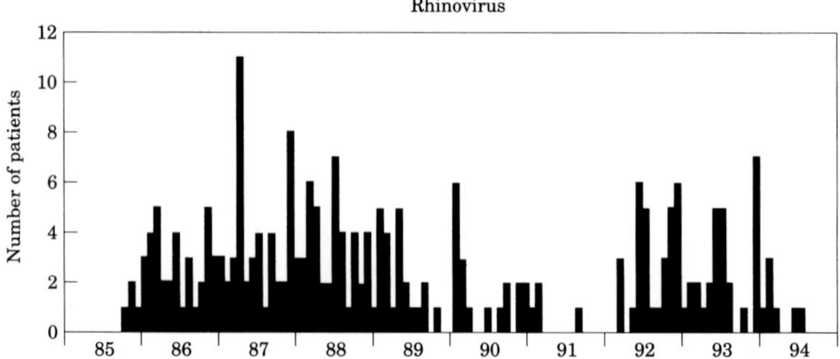

Fig 5.1 Incidence of adenoviruses and rhinoviruses isolated from children in the Royal Hospital for Sick Children, Edinburgh, October 1985–July 1994

Source: Reprinted from G. F. Winter et al (1996), with permission of W. B. Saunders Company Ltd

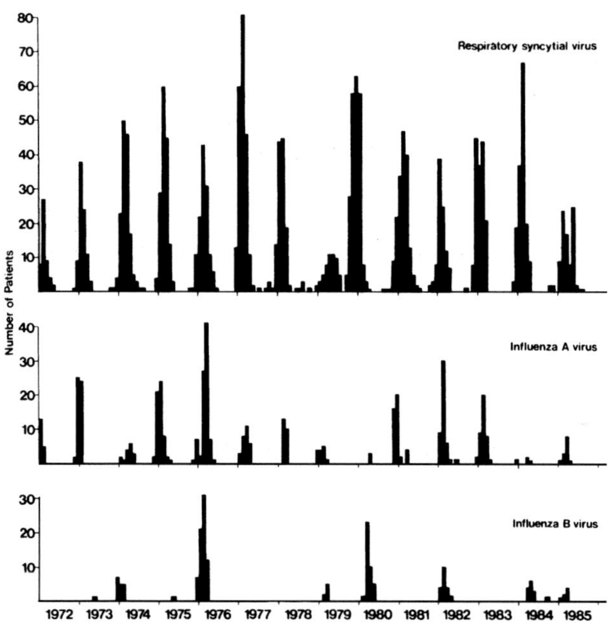

Fig 5.2 Incidence of respiratory syncytial and influenza A and B viruses detected in children in the Royal Hospital for Sick Children, Edinburgh, 1972–1985

Source: Reprinted from G. F. Winter and J. M. Inglis (1987), with permission of W. B. Saunders Company Ltd

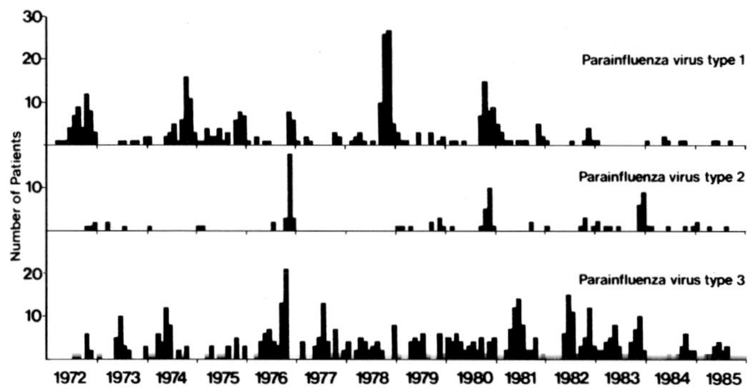

Fig 5.3 Incidence of parainfluenza virus types1, 2 and 3 isolated from children in the Royal Hospital for Sick Children, Edinburgh, 1972–1985

Source: Reprinted from G. F. Winter and J. M. Inglis (1987), with permission of W. B. Saunders Company Ltd

Respiratory viruses are associated with exacerbations of chronic bronchitis (McHardy et al, 1980) and asthma (Papadopoulos and Johnston, 1998), and can precipitate wheezing in children (Mitchell et al, 1978). The relatively recent discovery that respiratory viruses can cause serious infections in the immunocompromised (Bodey, 1997) underlines their continuing challenge to public health.

INFLUENZA VIRUSES

As coughs and colds raged around 15th-century Tuscany, feverish Florentines blamed the epidemic on the influence of the stars. They called it influenza. The great influenza pandemic of 1918–19 killed at least 20 million people worldwide, including at least 200,000 in England and Wales (Wiselka, 1994). In addition to the recent major pandemics of 1918–19, 1957, 1968 and 1977, regular epidemics occur worldwide with significant mortality, morbidity and economic loss.

Most of the influenza-related deaths which occur annually among the thousands of hospital admissions in the UK occur in those aged over 65 years. However, annual vaccination of the elderly helps to prevent morbidity and mortality (Diguiseppi, 1996).

The World Health Organisation maintains a global surveillance of influenza through a network of 108 National Influenza Centres in 76 countries. The aims of influenza surveillance are:

- to isolate circulating influenzaviruses and compare them with existing vaccine strains
- to monitor community spread of influenza and inform those concerned with disease control
- to determine how the impact of influenza outbreaks might influence the allocation of resources for appropriate control strategies

The family *Orthomyxoviridae* (Gr. *myxo* = mucus) contains the single genus influenzavirus, of which there are three members, A, B and C. Only type A causes widespread epidemics and has the potential to cause pandemics; type B is occasionally associated with epidemics of influenza; type C causes only very mild disease, if any. The surface of the influenza virus is covered with two types of glycoprotein spike, the more numerous haemagglutinin (H) and neuraminidase (N). H serves in the attachment of viruses to specific receptor sites on the surface of respiratory tract epithelial cells during the initial stages of infection; N is an enzyme thought to mediate the release of new viruses from the surface of infected cells. It is these projections which are largely responsible for the success of influenza.

H and N are the first parts of the virus encountered by the immune system, which produces specific antibodies to H and N; it is mainly the presence of an antibody to H which is protective. However, the influenza virus is unstable and makes mistakes as it copies its genes. If such errors are made, say while the H gene is copied, the H spikes will be altered. The resultant virus may elude antibodies raised against the original influenza virus. Minor changes in the configuration of the H and N spikes are called *antigenic drift* and account for new influenza outbreaks every year or so. Major, wholesale changes in spike configuration are called *antigenic shift*, and are responsible for influenza pandemics.

Influenza subtypes are classified according to the differences in H and N spikes. Thus, the pandemic of 1918 was caused by H1N1. This virus underwent antigenic drift until 1957 when H2N2, the Asian flu virus, replaced it. In 1968 Hong Kong flu kept the same N spike, but changed its H spike, becoming H3N2. However, a strain of H1N1, which had circulated in 1950, reappeared in 1977, surprising many researchers, and emphasising the capricious nature of influenza. Pigs, ducks and other waterfowl are important reservoirs of influenza, allowing viruses to mix, or reassort, from where they may infect humans. For example, 18 human cases of avian influenza H5N1 occurred in Hong Kong between May and December 1998, resulting in six deaths, raising fears of a new pandemic, and triggering a Phase 1 response of a pandemic preparedness plan (Dedman et al, 1998). But H5 is from chickens, the infected humans were end hosts, and the virus failed to spread from human to human, hence no pandemic occurred.

Respiratory syncytial virus

A member of the *Paramyxoviridae* family, RSV is the major respiratory pathogen of infants and young children, where it is usually manifested as pneumonia and bronchiolitis. In one study of respiratory viruses in a hospitalised population (Winter et al, 1996), more than half of the identified respiratory viruses were RSV, and almost 70% of respiratory infections occurred in children less than one year old (Table 5.1). RSV can repeatedly reinfect individuals throughout life and can infect infants who have maternal antibody. Although important as a paediatric pathogen, RSV can cause life-threatening pulmonary disease in the immunocompromised and the elderly. It causes annual epidemics of infection in temperate countries during the winter months (Winter and Inglis, 1987) and is highly contagious in all age groups (Hall, 1982), presenting considerable infection-control problems in hospitals (Doherty et al, 1998).

		Age (years)					M/F Ratio
Virus	**Total**	**<1**	**1–5**	**6–10**	**11–14**	**Unknown**	
Respiratory syncytial	1308	1071	197	13	4	23	1.4
Influenza A	87	31	43	9	3	1	1.3
Influenza B	48	19	19	9	1		1.3
Parainfluenza type 1	66						
Parainfluenza type 2	64	123	113	10		9	1.4
Parainfluenza type 3	125						
Rhino	239	157	66	9	3	4	1.3
Adeno	291	141	137	9	1	3	1.6
Total	2228	1542	575	59	12	40	Mean 1.37
(%)	(100)	(69.20)	(25.81)	(2.65)	(0.54)	(1.80)	

Table 5.1 Age and sex distribution of children in the Royal Hospital for Sick Children, Edinburgh, in whom respiratory viruses were identified, October 1985–July 1994

Source: Reprinted from G. F. Winter et al (1996), with permission of W. B. Saunders Company Ltd

RSV is spread via contaminated nasal secretions, with inoculation occurring mainly through the eye and nose, requiring close contact with an infected individual or a contaminated surface (Hall, 1982). Cohorting and handwashing are the best means of preventing the spread of RSV in hospital wards (Madeley, 1995). While the antiviral agent ribavirin has been useful in the clinical management of selected individual patients, one study found that vitamin A supplementation may have a role in the more general management of children infected with RSV (Neuzil et al, 1994).

The discovery of two subtypes of human RSV, subtype A and subtype B (Mufson et al, 1985), has allowed epidemiological studies of subtype variations during epidemics (Cane et al, 1994), and these subtypes must be considered when planning vaccine strategies. The aim of RSV vaccination is not to prevent RSV infection, but to prevent RSV-associated lower respiratory tract disease. Recently, two promising candidate RSV vaccines have been evaluated in clinical trials; one for immunising the elderly and older RSV-seropositive children with cardiac or pulmonary disease, and the other for immunising infants (Dudas and Karron, 1998).

Parainfluenza viruses

Parainfluenza (PIV) viruses types 1, 2, 3 and 4, which belong to the *Paramyxoviridae* family, are second only to RSV as the most important causes of serious respiratory infections in infants and young children; PIV type 3 is the most prevalent serotype, and one study (Glezen et al, 1984) found the risk for hospitalisation with PIV type 3 to be about one-fifth that for RSV infection. Croup is the commonest clinical manifestation of PIV infection in children (Downham et al, 1974; Knott et al, 1994), and a characteristic feature of PIVs is the high frequency of reinfections in both children and adults.

The pattern of PIV type 3 infection appears to have changed over the last 20 years from endemic to epidemic (Knott et al, 1994; Glezen et al, 1984). From the suggestion that two subtypes of PIV type 3 might exist (Hope-Simpson, 1981), it has been speculated that one subtype may spread optimally over a narrow temperature range to cause epidemic disease (de Silva and Cloonan, 1991).

Rhinoviruses

When the Medical Research Council's Common Cold Unit was founded after World War II, volunteers seeking a Club 18–50 holiday destination with a difference (Fig 5.4) could be seen walking in the rain, standing in draughty corridors wearing bathing costumes, and playing cards in rooms seeded with bumper packs of sneezing powder. Some of these seemingly bizarre experiments were used to establish that colds are not caused by chilling, changes in the weather or inadequate clothing. When the Unit closed in 1990, it had long been established that colds are caused not by one, but by a variety of different agents. However, rhinoviruses are the major causative agents of the common cold.

Would you like

TEN DAYS FREE HOLIDAY

and Travel Expenses paid?

All you have to do is to help the research into the common cold and influenza at the Research Centre in Salisbury, Wilts.

Over 400 people come every year but MORE ARE WANTED URGENTLY.

Comfortable accommodation for married or single people aged 18–50 years.

If interested write for details to:
COMMON COLD UNIT, SALISBURY, WILTS SP2 8BW

Fig 5.4 An advertisement from the Medical Research Council's Common Cold Unit

Source: Regional Clinical Virology Laboratory, City Hospital, Edinburgh EH10 5SB

Belonging to the *Picornaviridae* family, there are at least 115 serotypes of rhinovirus and they are the commonest viral cause of uncomplicated respiratory infections among children and adults. However, rhinoviruses can also be associated with serious respiratory tract illness (McMillan et al, 1993), and are the commonest viral initiators of wheeze in children (Mitchell et al, 1978).

Adenoviruses

Outbreaks of acute respiratory disease due to adenovirus infection can occur among military recruits, but are less common among healthy civilians. It is usually caused by adenovirus types 4, 7 and 21. In the USA, oral enteric-coated adenovirus vaccines have been used in the US Army to protect against adenovirus related acute respiratory disease.

In children under four years of age, adenoviruses account for 5% of acute respiratory infections and about 10% of hospitalised respiratory infections (Wadell, 1987). Although pharyngitis and associated tonsillitis and conjunctivitis are characteristic symptoms, adenovirus pneumonia is the most serious clinical manifestation in children, accounting for 10% of childhood pneumonias (Wadell, 1987).

Strains of adenovirus type 7 have been associated with severe disease and significant mortality (de Silva et al, 1989). In one nosocomial outbreak of adenovirus type 7 infection in a paediatric respiratory unit, 32 out of 207 children admitted during an eight-month period were infected with adenovirus, and of these 67% died (Wesley et al, 1993). Nosocomial spread was thought to be from attendants' hands, especially those handling suction catheters, endotracheal tubes or ventilator connections.

Coronaviruses

Human coronaviruses (HCV) were first isolated in the mid-1960s and infect all age groups, causing about 30% of common colds, with epidemic peaks generally occurring during the winter and early spring (Macnaughton, 1987). However, routine diagnostic laboratories seldom undertake HCV diagnosis because of complicated culture requirements. This, combined with their relatively minor clinical significance, accounts for the low virological profile of these agents.

Laboratory diagnosis

The rapid diagnosis of respiratory virus infections is especially important because of their short incubation periods and ease of spread, which may be global, as with influenza. The inoculation of respiratory specimens into cell-culture tubes, allied to the direct detection of viral antigen in cellular specimens have been the mainstay of the rapid laboratory diagnosis of respiratory virus infections for over 20 years.

The advent of the polymerase chain reaction (PCR) has seen many applications in pathology (O'Leary et al, 1997), and the evaluation of PCR techniques for respiratory viruses is currently underway. PCR should be helpful in the diagnosis of HCV infections, for which no simple, standard detection methods are available. However, further validation and standardisation of the PCR, as applied to respiratory viruses, is needed before it can progress beyond a research setting. The cost-effective use of pathology services demands that the introduction of relatively new techniques such as PCR can be justified on economic grounds (Halonen et al, 1996).

References

Bodey, G. P. (1997) Community respiratory viral infections in the immunocompromised host: past, present, and future directions. *American Journal of Medicine*; 102: (3A), 77–80.

Cane, P. A., Matthews, D. A., Pringle, C. R. (1994) Analysis of respiratory syncytial virus strain variation in successive epidemics in one city. *Journal of Clinical Microbiology*; 32: 1, 1–4.

Dedman, D. J., Zambon, M., Van Buynder, P. et al (1998) Influenza surveillance in England and Wales: October 1997 to June 1998. *Communicable Disease and Public Health*; 1: 4, 244–251.

de Silva, L. M., Colditz, P., Wadell, G. (1989) Adenovirus type 7 infections in children in New South Wales, Australia. *Journal of Medical Virology*; 29: 28–32.

de Silva, L. M., Cloonan, M. J. (1991) Brief report: parainfluenza virus type 3 infections: findings in Sydney and some observations on variations in seasonality world-wide. *Journal of Medical Virology*; 35: 19–21.

Diguiseppi, C. (1996) Why everyone over 65 deserves influenza vaccine. *British Medical Journal*; 313: 1162.

Doherty, J. A., Brookfield, D. S. K., Gray, J., McEwan, R.A. (1998) Cohorting of infants with respiratory syncytial virus. *Journal of Hospital Infection*; 38: 203–206.

Downham, M. A. P. S., McQuillin, J., Gardner, P. S. (1974) Diagnosis and clinical significance of parainfluenza virus infections in children. *Archives of Disease in Childhood*; 49: 8–15.

Dudas, R. A., Karron, R. A. (1998) Respiratory syncytial virus vaccines. *Clinical Microbiolgy Reviews*; 11: 3, 430–439.

Glezen, W. P., Frank, A. L., Taber, L. H., Kasel, J. A. (1984) Parainfluenza type 3: seasonality and risk of infection and reinfection in young children. *Journal of Infectious Diseases*; 150: 6, 851–857.

Hall, C. B. (1982) Respiratory syncytial virus: its transmission in the hospital environment. *Yale Journal of Biology and Medicine*; 55: 219–223.

Halonen, P., Hierholzer, J., Ziegler, T. (1996) Advances in the diagnosis of respiratory virus infections. *Clinical and Diagnostic Virology*; 5: 2/3, 91–100.

Hope-Simpson, R. E. (1981) Parainfluenza virus infections in the Cirencester Survey: seasonal and other characteristics. *Journal of Hygiene, Cambridge*; 87: 393–406.

Knott, A. M., Long, C. E., Hall, C. B. (1994) Parainfluenza viral infections in pediatric outpatients: seasonal patterns and clinical characteristics. *Pediatric Infectious Disease Journal*; 13: 4, 269–273.

McHardy, V. U., Inglis, J. M., Calder, M. A., Crofton, J. W. (1980) A study of infective and other factors in exacerbations of chronic bronchitis. *British Journal of Diseases of the Chest*; 74: 228–238.

McMillan, J. A., Weiner, L. B., Higgins, A. M., Macknight, K. (1993) Rhinovirus infection associated with serious illness among pediatric patients. *Pediatric Infectious Disease Journal*; 12: 4, 321–325.

Macnaughton, M. R. (1987) Coronaviruses. In: Zuckerman, A. J., Banatvala, J. E., Pattison, J. R. (eds) *Principles and Practice of Clinical Virology*. Chichester: John Wiley & Sons.

Madeley, C. R. (1995) Viral infections in children's wards – how well do we manage them? *Journal of Hospital Infection*; 30: suppl., 163–171.

Mims, C. A. (1987) *The Pathogenesis of Infectious Disease*. London: Academic Press, 3rd edn.

Mitchell, I., Inglis, J. M., Simpson, H. (1978) Viral infection as a precipitant of wheeze in children: combined home and hospital study. *Archives of Disease in Childhood*; 53: 2, 106–111.

Mufson, M. A., Orvell, C., Rafnar, B., Norrby, E. (1985) Two distinct subtypes of human respiratory syncytial virus. *Journal of General Virology*; 66: 2111–2124.

Neuzil, K. M., Gruber, W. C., Chytil, F. et al (1994) Serum vitamin A levels in respiratory syncytial virus infection. *Journal of Paediatrics*; 124: 433–436.

O'Leary, J. J., Engels, K., Dada, M. A. (1997) The polymerase chain reaction in pathology. *Journal of Clinical Pathology*; 50: 10, 805–810.

Papadopoulos, N. G., Johnston, S. L. (1998) Viruses and asthma exacerbations. *Thorax*; 53: 11, 913–914.

Wadell, G. (1987) Adenoviruses. In: Zuckerman, A. J., Banatvala, J. E., Pattison, J.R. (eds) *Principles and Practice of Clinical Virology*. Chichester: John Wiley & Sons.

Wesley, A. G., Pather, M., Tait, D. (1993) Nosocomial adenovirus infection in a paediatric respiratory unit. *Journal of Hospital Infection*; 25: 183–190.

Winter, G. F., Inglis, J. M. (1987) Respiratory viruses in children admitted to hospital in Edinburgh 1972–85. *Journal of Infection*; 15: 103–107.

Winter, G. F., Hallam, N. F., Hargreaves, F. D. et al (1996) Respiratory viruses in a hospitalised paediatric population in Edinburgh 1985–1994. *Journal of Infection*; 33: 207–211.

Wiselka, M. (1994) Influenza: diagnosis, management, and prophylaxis. *British Medical Journal*; 308: 1341–1345.

6 The gastrointestinal tract

An immense slackening ache,
As when, thawing, the rigid landscape weeps,
Spreads slowly through them ...

Philip Larkin (1922–1985), 'Faith Healing'.

There is no doubt about it; it's rough down there. With acids, bile salts and the full panoply of digestive enzymes waiting to attack whatever is swallowed, we can safely assume that viruses associated with gastrointestinal infection are equipped to withstand the extremes of a physically and chemically hostile environment. But to compensate, they will find a rich source of constantly renewed cells being produced at a constant temperature, which provide many possibilities for infection.

Gastrointestinal infections are acquired by the faecal–oral route; viruses shed in faeces end up in someone else's mouth, either through food or water. Food can become contaminated by the unwashed hands of food handlers, by the use of human faeces as a soil fertiliser, or by flies. The water supply may become contaminated with inadequately treated sewage, and sewage-contaminated coastal waters pose a risk to bathers, wind-surfers and the like. The faecal–oral route of spread is favoured by insanitary living conditions such as those found in many developing countries, the socially deprived areas of developed countries and, for example, in some mental institutions. In addition, vomitus, droplets, and faecally contaminated fomites contribute to the transmission of stool viruses.

There are certain 'opportunistic' viruses whose presence in the gut is often the result of infection in immunocompromised individuals, and which are not acquired by the faecal–oral route. For example, herpes simplex virus (HSV) can cause proctitis, especially in male homosexuals; cytomegalovirus (CMV) can cause oesophagitis, gastritis, duodenitis and proctitis; certain human papillomaviruses (HPV) are associated with anal cancer; human immunodeficiency virus (HIV) is associated with chronic diarrhoea and malabsorption (Farthing, 1989).

It is something of a paradox that many viruses can be grown from faeces in cell culture, yet seldom cause disease in the gut. On the other hand, many viruses which *do* cause gastrointestinal upset cannot be easily grown in cell culture, and have been increasingly identified only since the 1970s. The advent of cell-culture techniques for virus cultivation ushered in what some call the 'golden age' of virology in the 1950s, when many new viruses were discovered.

Viruses grown from faeces

Viruses that can be grown from faeces belong to one of three groups:

- reoviruses
- adenoviruses
- enteroviruses

In 1959 Albert Sabin, who produced the first live poliomyelitis vaccine, gave the name reovirus to isolates of a ribonucleic acid (RNA) virus from faeces and rectal swabs which produced a characteristic cytopathic effect (CPE) in monkey-kidney cell cultures, and were pathogenic when injected into newborn mice (Tyler and Fields, 1996). The name denoted *r*espiratory *e*nteric *o*rphan viruses, as they could be isolated from respiratory and enteric specimens and did not seem to be associated with any 'parent' disease. Forty years later it is still the case that reoviruses have not been shown to produce any human diseases, although 'associations' abound, from upper respiratory infections to neonatal hepatitis to myocarditis (Tyler and Fields, 1996).

Adenoviruses were first isolated in 1953 from cultures of adenoidal tissue surgically removed from children. At first, some of these deoxyribonucleic acid (DNA) viruses were found to grow easily in the intestine and could be isolated from faeces, and it was assumed that adenoviruses were a likely cause of diarrhoea. However, it was then found that cultivable adenoviruses could be excreted by normal children. As we shall see, it is the adenoviruses which *cannot* be easily grown which cause most gastrointestinal upset, especially in children.

The enteroviruses, which belong to the *Picornaviridae* (small RNA viruses), are the largest group of viruses which can be grown from faeces. They include poliovirus (three serotypes), Coxsackie A virus (23 serotypes), Coxsackie B virus (six serotypes), *e*nteric *c*ytopathogenic *h*uman *o*rphan or echovirus (30 serotypes) and human enteroviruses 68–71 serotypes. Although most enterovirus infections are asymptomatic, they are, none the less, associated with a range of symptoms from mild respiratory disease to central nervous system (CNS) involvement with paralysis. Children have an important role in transmission, with inapparent excretion common, and are infected more often than adults (Grandien et al, 1995).

Because of the ravages of paralytic poliomyelitis, poliovirus has been the most intensively studied of the enteroviruses. Poliovirus infection can have one of four possible outcomes; inapparent infection, mild illness, aseptic meningitis, or paralytic poliomyelitis (Brooks et al, 1991), with only about 1% of poliovirus infections causing clinical disease (Melnick, 1996). In 1998 the UK Panel for the Certification of Elimination of Poliomyelitis submitted documentation to the World Health Organisation which would allow the UK to be declared free from poliomyelitis by the end of 1998 (*CDR Weekly*, 1998a), and it is hoped that global eradication will be achieved by 2005 (Finn and Bell, 1998).

The Coxsackie and echoviruses produce a variety of illnesses in man, including aseptic meningitis, acute haemorrhagic conjunctivitis, and mild febrile disease which occurs during the summer or autumn. Although a number of studies have indicated a possible role for Coxsackie B viruses in insulin-dependent diabetes mellitus, convincing evidence is awaited (Melnick, 1996). However, Coxsackie B viruses are the commonest cause of viral heart disease in humans (Brooks et al, 1991). Hand, foot and mouth disease (HFMD), a vesicular rash of the palms and soles with oral and pharyngeal ulceration, is mainly associated with Coxsackie A virus type 16, with death a very rare outcome. However, during April–July 1998 an outbreak of HFMD associated with enterovirus type 71 infection occurred among children in Taiwan, Republic of China (Centers for Disease Control and Prevention, 1998). Of 90,000 reported cases, 320 children were hospitalised, and at least 55 died. In the UK between the late 1950s and early 1990s, of the reported non-polio enterovirus infections, 61% were echoviruses, 30% Coxsackie B viruses and 9% Coxsackie A viruses, with echovirus type 11 particularly associated with neonatal infections (Hill, 1996).

The application of cell-culture techniques demonstrated the diversity of viruses which could be found in faeces. Yet despite this, the fact remained that few of them could be shown to be common causes of diarrhoea. When it was considered that bacterial pathogens were absent in more than 60% of patients with diarrhoea, it seemed that other, non-cultivable viruses could be involved. Indeed they were, but their discovery would have to wait until the 1970s, when electron microscopy (EM) was used for the direct examination of human faeces (Madeley, 1979).

Viruses detected by electron microscopy

It is, perhaps, surprising that we had to wait until 1972 for the demonstration of a virus as a cause of acute gastroenteritis in humans. As long ago as 1949 it had been shown that a filterable agent in faeces from newborn children could transmit diarrhoea to young calves. A series of studies throughout the 1950s and 1960s featured adult volunteers who were evidently agreeable to ingesting bacteria-free faecal filtrates from cases of acute gastroenteritis, in order to demonstrate the transmissibility of the presumed viral agents. These studies helped to establish the term 'acute non-bacterial gastroenteritis', but the identity of the agent(s) remained a mystery.

In October 1968, half of the students and teachers at a school in Norwalk, Ohio, USA, developed acute gastroenteritis. In 1972 Norwalk virus was identified by EM in faeces samples from the outbreak (Kapikian et al, 1972). In April 1973 Ruth Bishop and her colleagues used EM to detect rotaviruses in ultra-thin sections of duodenal epithelium from a child with acute gastroenteritis (Bishop et al, 1973). Many investigators now focused on faeces; astroviruses were first described in 1975 (Madeley and Cosgrove, 1975), human caliciviruses in 1976 (Madeley and Cosgrove, 1976), and small round viruses, 'fastidious' adenoviruses and coronaviruses have been detected by EM, and added to the list of viruses causing gastrointestinal upset.

Norwalk virus belongs to a group called small round-structured viruses (SRSV), which are the most common cause of outbreaks of gastrointestinal illness in the UK (Hale, 1997), responsible for 90% of food-related gastroenteritis outbreaks (PHLS Working Party, 1988). SRSVs are RNA viruses in the *Caliciviridae* family, have a worldwide distribution, primarily affect adults and school-age children, but do not appear to produce severe diarrhoea among infants and young children (Kapikian et al, 1996). Outbreaks tend to occur in schools, camps, institutions and the like, affecting large numbers of people within one or two days. For example, it was not such a *bon voyage* in April 1998, shortly after a cruise ship set sail from the Dominican Republic, and 347 passengers and 28 members of the crew reported a sudden onset of explosive diarrhoea and vomiting. SRSVs were detected by the polymerase chain reaction (PCR) on faeces samples from three passengers (*CDR Weekly*, 1998b). Although EM is still the routine diagnostic test of choice, the more sensitive PCR can be applied in research, and in the identification of SRSVs in shellfish, sewage and contaminated water (Hale, 1997).

Human caliciviruses (HuCV), belong to the same *Caliciviridae* family as SRSVs, but have a different appearance by EM. However, the clinical features, incubation period, and duration of symptoms are the same for HuCV as SRSVs (Cubitt, 1989). In the UK outbreaks of HuCV affecting all age groups have been recorded since 1978, with diarrhoea and vomiting the main features, often accompanied by abdominal pain in older children and adults (Cubitt, 1989).

Viral gastroenteritis can be either epidemic or sporadic. The former is most often associated with SRSVs and HuCV, and is seldom a cause for hospitalisation. However, sporadic viral gastroenteritis, most often associated with rotavirus (Fig 6.1), differs from the epidemic form by primarily affecting those under two years of age, and by having a range of outcomes from subclinical infection to life-threatening illness (Kapikian, 1993).

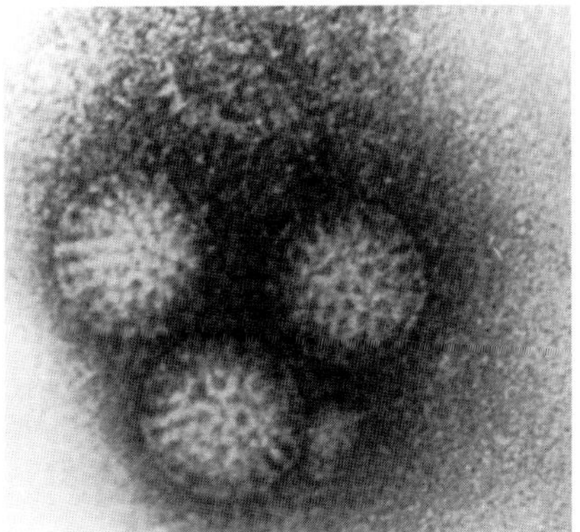

Fig 6.1 Rotavirus in faeces from a neonate with acute diarrhoea and vomiting
Source: Courtesy of Dr W. D. Cubitt, Great Ormond Street Hospital for Children NHS Trust, London WC1N 3JH

Globally, rotaviruses are the single most important cause of diarrhoea in young children, causing acute diarrhoea in about 40% of children requiring hospitalisation in developing countries and in 50%–60% of children admitted to hospital in developed countries (Bishop, 1984). In the context of between 3 and 6 million children dying annually from diarrhoeal illness (Thielman et al, 1996), rotavirus represents a considerable problem, especially in the Third World. However, the application of appropriate, simple oral rehydration therapy saves many lives by reversing the massive net secretion of electrolytes and water.

Rotavirus infection in adults is often asymptomatic, although young adults and elderly patients can experience severe symptoms. However, while all age groups can be affected, children under two years of age are especially vulnerable to serious diarrhoeal illness caused by rotaviruses, and in developing countries infant mortality is high. According to Ryder et al (cited by Herrmann and Blacklow, 1995), about 20% of rotavirus infections in hospital are nosocomial, which presents a considerable infection-control challenge. This, in turn, requires prompt laboratory diagnosis, and EM can give quick results, although it is relatively insensitive. However, the availability of commercial diagnostic kits and techniques, such as polyacrylamide gel electrophoresis, mean that timely laboratory diagnosis of rotavirus infection is possible, allowing appropriate infection-control measures to be taken. Meanwhile, there are hopes for an effective rotavirus vaccine which would prevent rotavirus gastroenteritis during the first two years of life. For instance, it is estimated that rotavirus vaccination in developing countries could save at least 500,000 deaths each year (Vesikari, 1989), and a recent study in Finland showed that a live, attenuated rotavirus vaccine could reduce severe gastroenteritis in young children by 90%; the authors believe that the results support the introduction of rotavirus vaccination into childhood immunisation programmes, subject to cost-benefit analyses in each country (Joensuu et al, 1997). However, the economic constraints in developing countries are such that a vaccine from the developed world may be too expensive for use among the populations most in need in the developing world. Some feel that with the scientific challenge of rotavirus vaccination almost solved, a greater moral challenge remains (Keusch and Cash, 1997).

Many adenoviruses replicate easily in the gut, and can be detected in the faeces of normal and diarrhoeic children, which has made it difficult to define the role of these viruses in gastroenteritis. However, two adenovirus types were identified which could be seen by EM, but which failed to grow in routine cell cultures. Thus adenovirus types 40 and 41, the so-called 'non-cultivable' or 'fastidious' adenoviruses, have been consistently associated with infantile gastroenteritis, responsible for between 5% and 10% of all cases. The enteric adenoviruses are the second most important viral cause of endemic diarrhoea in young children worldwide (Kapikian, 1993). In a recent UK study of 452 faeces samples from children with gastroenteritis found by EM to contain adenovirus, 22% contained adenovirus type 40, 46% adenovirus type 41 and 32% other adenovirus types (Bryden et al, 1997). The incubation period of 8–10 days compares with 1–3 days for rotavirus and Norwalk virus.

In 1975 human astroviruses were first observed by EM in the faeces of infants hospitalised with gastroenteritis (Madeley and Cosgrove, 1975). They are RNA viruses with a characteristic star-like appearance, belonging to the *Astroviridae* family, which primarily affect young children worldwide. In a study involving 3,150 Thai children (Herrmann et al, 1991), it was found that astroviruses are important agents of gastroenteritis, with clinical findings closely matching those of rotavirus. Surprisingly, in this study they found that astroviruses were associated with illness more often than enteric adenoviruses.

We can speculate that new infectious causes of gastroenteritis have yet to be found. Over the last 25 years or so, viruses and virus-like particles have been seen in human faeces by EM. For example, at a school in the Australian city of Parramatta, parvovirus-like particles were seen in 14 faeces samples examined during an outbreak of acute gastroenteritis, which affected 217 individuals (Christopher et al, 1978), and particles resembling orthomyxoviruses and coronaviruses were seen in faeces samples of south Indian adults and children with and without gastrointestinal illness (Mathan et al, 1973).

Clearly, further studies are required to clarify the role(s) if any of, as yet, poorly defined viruses or virus-like particles seen in human faeces by EM. One group of viruses, not yet mentioned, can occasionally complicate matters for electron microscopists: the bacteriophages. These are viruses which infect bacteria, but not human cells. Nevertheless, they serve to emphasise that not everything which is seen by EM and looks like a virus in the faeces is necessarily important in terms of human disease.

References

Bishop, R. F., Davidson, G. P., Holmes, I. H., Ruck, B. J. (1973) Virus particles in epithelial cells of duodenal mucosa from children with acute gastroenteritis. *Lancet*; 2: 1281–1283.

Bishop, R. F. (1984) Rotavirus in perspective – a personal view. *Australian Paediatric Journal*; 20: 9–12.

Brooks, G. F., Butel, J. S., Ornston, L. N. (1991) Picornaviruses (enterovirus and rhinovirus groups). In: *Jawetz, Melnick and Adelberg's Medical Microbiology*. East Norwalk, CT: Appleton & Lange.

Bryden, A. S., Curry, A., Cotterill, H. et al (1997) Adenovirus-associated gastroenteritis in the north-west of England:1991–1994. *British Journal of Biomedical Science*; 54: 273–277.

CDR Weekly (1998a) Acute flaccid paralysis and the eradication of poliomyelitis; 8: 17, 147–150.

CDR Weekly (1998b) An outbreak of viral gastroenteritis on board a cruise liner; 8: 17, 147.

Centers for Disease Control and Prevention (1998). Deaths among children during an outbreak of Hand, Foot, and Mouth Disease – Taiwan, Republic of China, April–July 1998. *Morbidity and Mortality Weekly Report*; 47: 30, 629–632.

Christopher, P. J., Grohmann, G. S., Millsom, R. H., Murphy, A. M. (1978) Parvovirus gastroenteritis – a new entity for Australia. *Medical Journal of Australia*; 1: 3, 121–124.

Cubitt, W. D. (1989) Diagnosis, occurrence and clinical significance of the human 'candidate' caliciviruses. *Progress in Medical Virology*; 36: 103–119.

Farthing, M. J. G. (1989) Gut viruses: a role in gastrointestinal disease? In: *Viruses and the Gut. Proceedings of the Ninth BSG.SK and F International Workshop 1988.* Welwyn Garden City: Smith Kline & French Laboratories.

Finn, A., Bell, F. (1998) Polio vaccine: is it time for a change? *Archives of Disease in Childhood*; 78: 571–574.

Grandien, M., Forsgren, M., Ehrnst, A. (1995) Enteroviruses. In: Lennette, E. H., Lennette, D. A., Lennette, E. T. (eds) *Diagnostic Procedures for Viral, Rickettsial, and Chlamydial Infections*, Washington: American Public Health Association, 7th edn.

Hale, A. D. (1997) Recent advances in the diagnosis of small round structured viruses. *Reviews in Medical Microbiology*; 8: 3, 149–155.

Herrmann, J. E., Blacklow, N. R. (1995) Gastroenteritis viruses. In: Lennette, E. H., Lennette, D. A., Lennette, E. T. (eds) *Diagnostic Procedures for Viral, Rickettsial, and Chlamydial Infections*. Washington: American Public Health Association, 7th edn.

Herrmann, J. E., Taylor, D. N., Echeverria, P., Blacklow, N. R. (1991) Astroviruses as a cause of gastroenteritis in children. *New England Journal of Medicine*; 324: 25, 1757–1760.

Hill, W. M. J. (1996) Are echoviruses still orphans? *British Journal of Biomedical Science*; 53: 221–226.

Joensuu, J., Koskenniemi, E., Pang, X., Vesikari, T. (1997) Randomised placebo-controlled trial of rhesus-human reassortant rotavirus vaccine for prevention of severe rotavirus gastroenteritis. *Lancet*; 350: 1205–1209.

Kapikian, A. Z., Wyatt, R. G., Dolin, R. et al (1972) Visualisation by immune electron microscopy of a 27-nm particle associated with acute infectious nonbacterial gastroenteritis. *Journal of Virology*; 10: 1075–1081.

Kapikian, A. Z. (1993) Viral gastroenteritis. *Journal of the American Medical Association*; 269: 5, 627–630.

Kapikian, A. Z., Estes, M. K., Chanock, R. M. (1996) Norwalk Group of Viruses. In: Fields, B. N., Knipe, D. M., Howley, P. M. et al (eds) *Fields Virology*, Philadelphia: Lippincott-Raven, 3rd edn.

Keusch, G. T., Cash, R. A. (1997) A vaccine against rotavirus – when is too much too much? *New England Journal of Medicine*; 337: 17, 1228–1229.

Madeley, C. R. (1979) Viruses in the stools. *Journal of Clinical Pathology*; 32: 1–10.

Madeley, C. R., Cosgrove, B. P. (1975) 28nm particles in faeces in infantile gastroenteritis. *Lancet*; 2: 451–452.

Madeley, C. R., Cosgrove, B. P. (1976) Caliciviruses in man. *Lancet*; 1: 199.

Mathan, M., Mathan,V. I., Swaminathan, S. P. et al (1973) Pleomorphic virus-like particles in human faeces. *Lancet*; 1: 1068–1069.

Melnick, J. L. (1996) Enteroviruses: polioviruses, coxsackieviruses, echoviruses, and newer enteroviruses. In: Fields, B. N., Knipe, D. M., Howley, P. M. et al (eds) *Fields Virology*. Philadelphia: Lippincott-Raven, 3rd edn.

PHLS Working Party on Viral Gastroenteritis (1988) Foodborne viral gastroenteritis: an overview (with a brief comment on hepatitis A). *PHLS Microbiology Digest*; 5: 69–75.

Thielman, N. M., Guerrant, R. L. (1996) From Rwanda to Wisconsin: the global relevance of diarrhoeal diseases. *Journal of Medical Microbiology*; 44: 155–156.

Tyler, K. L., Fields, B. N. (1996) Reoviruses. In: Fields, B. N., Knipe, D. M., Howley, P. M. et al (eds) *Fields Virology*. Philadelphia: Lippincott-Raven, 3rd edn.

Vesikari, T. (1989) Clinical trials of rotavirus vaccines. In: *Viruses and the Gut. Proceedings of the Ninth BSG.SK and F International Workshop 1988.* Welwyn Garden City: Smith Kline & French Laboratories.

7 The skin

That, my friend, is all there is
Between you and the abyss.
Two hundred and nineteen square inches of Goddamn skin!

George A. Ferguson (1914–), 'O Jesus! O Epidermis!'

Weighing in at roughly 5kg, and with an area of around 1.75 square metres, the skin presents a relatively impermeable, and sometimes hairy, barrier to the environment, hosting a diversity of flora and fauna, some of which are pathogenic, many of which are not. Far from being inert, the skin's surface is being constantly worn away and replaced with new cells pushed up from the basal cell layer of the epidermis. This epidermal 'turnover' time has been variously estimated at between 14 and 45 days (Noble, 1981).

Breaches in the integrity of the skin clearly invite infection. For example, hepatitis B virus (HBV) can typically be acquired through the skin being punctured by the contaminated needle of a tattooist, body-piercer or drug abuser. Dengue, the most important arthropod-borne viral disease of humans (Monath, 1995), is introduced directly into the bloodstream through a mosquito bite. In rabies the disease is commonly transmitted by the bite of a mammal.

The skin and contiguous mucous membranes can be the site of localised virus infections, resulting in warts, for example. Alternatively, the skin may be the organ in which systemic disease first becomes apparent, usually by way of a characteristic rash. For example, in measles the virus is found in the blood vessels of the skin, but the maculopapular rash is dependent on an adequate immune response being mounted. Yet other viruses, such as varicella zoster virus (VZV), may spread from dermal blood vessels into superficial skin layers to form vesicles or pustules.

Poxviruses

The family *Poxviridae* are the largest human viruses, brick-shaped, with a complex coat enclosing a deoxyribonucleic acid (DNA) genome.

On 26 October 1979 the World Health Organisation declared the world free of smallpox, a virus which has killed more people than any other infectious disease, and in May 1996, the World Health Assembly resolved that the remaining laboratory stocks of variola virus should be destroyed on 30 June 1999 (Ellner, 1998). Variola, the cause of smallpox, was eliminated through vaccination with vaccinia virus, a poxvirus whose origins are obscure.

During the closing stages of the smallpox eradication campaign, monkeypox posed some diagnostic problems. In monkeys the virus produces a mild illness with a vesicular rash, and when transmitted to man, monkeypox produces an illness similar to mild smallpox.

Other poxvirus infections of man may be found down on the farm. Cowpox virus produces lesions on the hands, arms or face of humans in contact with infected cows, although some individuals may have had no direct contact with cows or carcasses. Lesions begin as papules which become vesicular and then pustular. The virus causing milkers' node is often transmitted from infected cows' udders to the hands of milkers, and occasionally indirectly transmitted to dairy workers, veterinary surgeons or butchers. Orf is commonly found in young lambs worldwide, and the virus is transmitted by direct inoculation to the hands, forearms or face of shepherds, veterinary surgeons and allied workers (Fig 7.1). Papules develop into haemorrhagic pustules which often have a central depression. Cowpox, milkers' node and orf usually heal spontaneously within six weeks (Robinson and Heath, 1983a).

Molluscum contagiosum is a benign, self-limiting skin tumour caused by a poxvirus affecting only humans. The lesions are pearly, raised nodules, about 2–5mm in diameter (Fig 7.2). The disease is found worldwide, occurring sporadically, or causing epidemics in institutions where spread is influenced by poor hygiene, poverty and overcrowding (Postlethwaite, 1970). In children molluscum contagiosum virus (MCV) is transmitted by direct skin contact and by fomites, with boys more susceptible than girls. In adults tattooing, wrestling and shared clothing account for some of the non-sexual modes of transmission of MCV. However, sexual transmission of MCV is increasingly common. For example, 5,053 cases of molluscum contagiosum were diagnosed at genitourinary medicine clinics in England in 1996, an increase of 13% over the previous year (Simms et al, 1998). Genital MCV infection may be a marker for other sexually transmitted diseases and for human immunodeficiency virus (HIV) infection, and molluscum contagiosum is relatively common among AIDS patients, and is associated with other immunosuppressive states (Birthistle and Carrington, 1997).

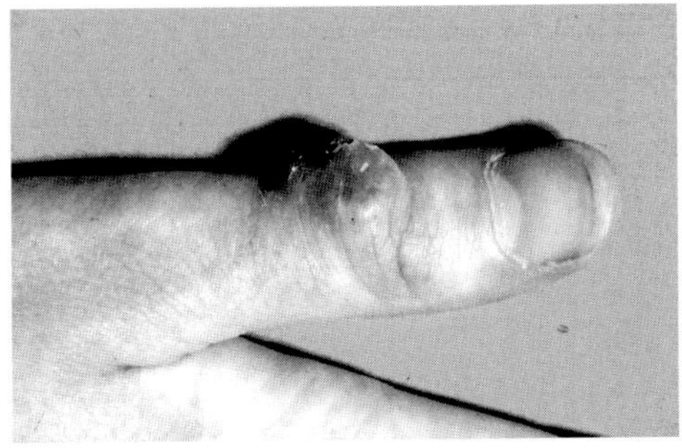

Fig 7.1 A human orf lesion
Source: Courtesy of Professor A. Nash, University of Glasgow Veterinary School, Glasgow G61 1QH

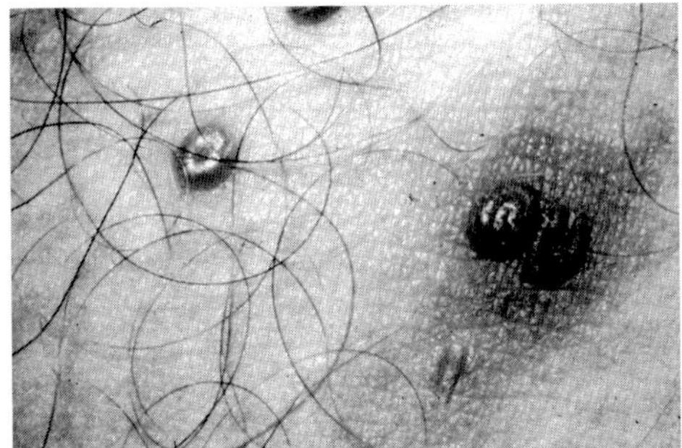

Fig 7.2 Molluscum contagiosum lesions
Source: Courtesy of Dr Sheila M. Burns, Regional Clinical Virology Laboratory, City Hospital, Edinburgh EH10 5SB

HERPESVIRUSES

The *Herpesviridae* family contains eight human herpesviruses, many of which produce skin manifestations in addition to systemic disease. The main biological feature of herpesviruses is that they remain latent in their natural hosts, but may reactivate to produce recurrent disease.

Herpes simplex virus (HSV) infections are acquired through contaminated secretions during close personal contact. There are two types of HSV; type 1 and type 2. In general, HSV-1 causes more infections above the waist than HSV-2, which is mainly associated with genital infection. Both types can cause primary and recurrent infections.

Fig 7.3 Herpes simplex stomatitis
Source: Courtesy of Dr Sheila M. Burns, Regional Clinical Virology Laboratory, City Hospital, Edinburgh EH10 5SB

In infants and children the most common clinical outcome of primary HSV-1 infection is acute gingivostomatitis (Fig 7.3), mainly affecting the mucous membranes, whereas in adults, primary HSV-1 infection is often associated with acute upper respiratory tract infection. Skin lesions associated with primary HSV-1 infection include:

- primary herpetic dermatitis, usually seen in young children, where the rash may resemble chickenpox
- traumatic herpes, where virus enters directly through a break in the skin, as in herpetic whitlows (Fig 7.4)

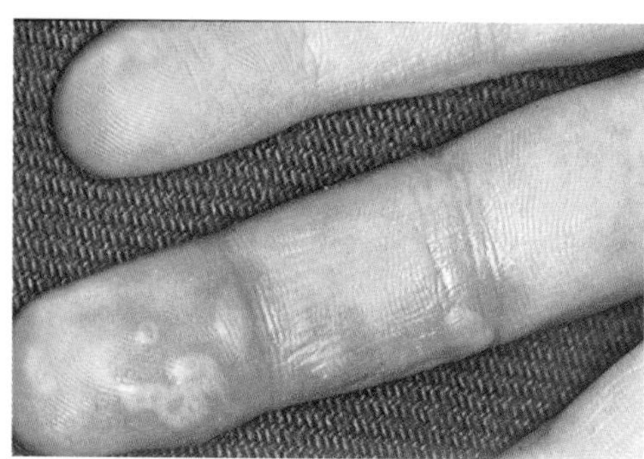

Fig 7.4 Herpetic whitlow
Source: Courtesy of Dr Sheila M. Burns, Regional Clinical Virology Laboratory, City Hospital, Edinburgh EH10 5SB

- eczema herpeticum, a severe infection often seen in patients with atopic eczema

In adults primary infection with HSV-2 may result in genital herpes (Fig 7.5). Although HSV-2 is isolated more often than HSV-1, both types cause primary genital herpes. However, HSV-2 is seen more often in male homosexuals (Carrington, 1996). Neonatal HSV infection is usually acquired at delivery, and HSV-2 causes more than 80% of cases, with the outcome ranging from virtually asymptomatic infection to severe fulminating disease which can be fatal if untreated. In about one-third of these cases, a vesicular skin rash occurs which may involve the mouth, eyes and mucous membranes (Robinson and Heath, 1983b).

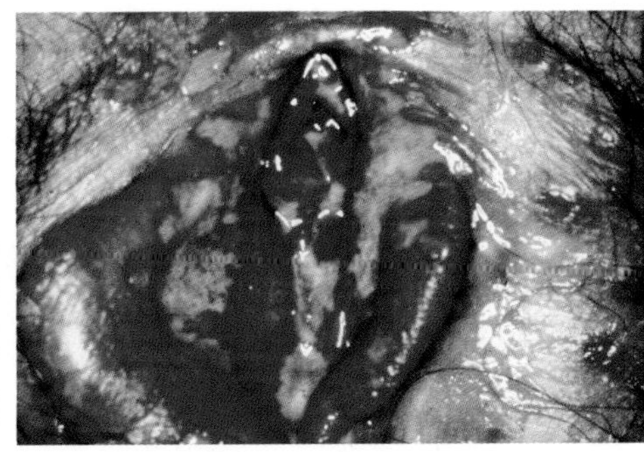

Fig 7.5 Genital herpes simplex infection in a female
Source: Courtesy of Dr Sheila M. Burns, Regional Clinical Virology Laboratory, City Hospital, Edinburgh EH10 5SB

It has been estimated that about one-third of those living in industrialised countries have cold sores (WHO Meeting, 1985), and those afflicted readers will confirm that HSV infections can recur. Recurrences happen because of the phenomenon of latency.

During the course of viral multiplication at the point of entry into the body, HSV infects the nerve endings and travels up to the dorsal root ganglia, where it remains latent in the neurons. Under physical and/or emotional stress the latent virus becomes activated, and travels via the axon to the original point of entry, where it may cause a lesion. In HSV-1 infection, following stomatitis, for example, the virus remains latent in the trigeminal or superior cervical ganglia, whereas following genital infection with HSV-2, the virus usually remains latent in the sacral ganglion. Latent virus is shielded from the immune system and represents a potentially infectious reservoir, probably accounting for the widespread dissemination of HSV in human populations.

Varicella zoster virus (VZV) causes varicella, or chickenpox; and herpes zoster, or shingles (Figs 7.6 and 7.7). After primary infection, VZV becomes latent in the cells of the dorsal root ganglia. Herpes zoster is caused by reactivation of VZV, often many years later, and the incidence of herpes zoster increases with age or immunosuppression. Shingles cannot be 'caught' from contact with a case of chickenpox.

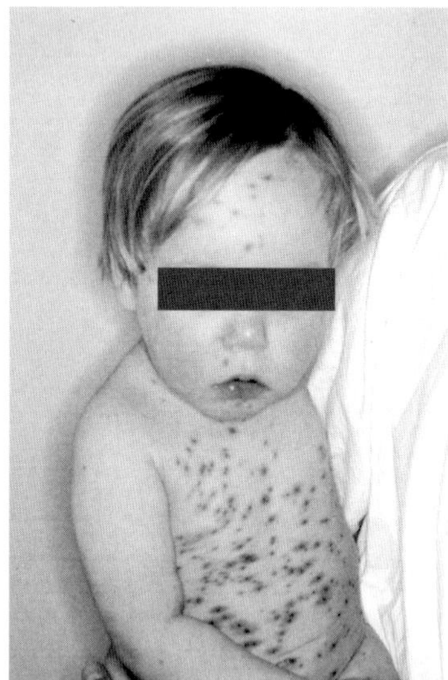

Fig 7.6 Varicella, or chickenpox
Source: Courtesy of Dr Sheila M. Burns, Regional Clinical Virology Laboratory, City Hospital, Edinburgh EH10 5SB

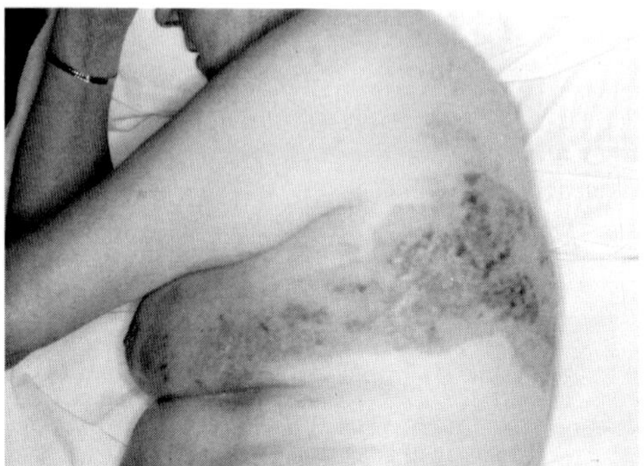

Fig 7.7 Herpes zoster, or shingles
Source: Courtesy of Dr Sheila M. Burns, Regional Clinical Virology Laboratory, City Hospital, Edinburgh EH10 5SB

Unlike herpes zoster, which has no seasonal pattern (Arvin, 1996), chickenpox is most prevalent in winter and spring months and is highly contagious, with transmission usually by the respiratory route. The incubation period of chickenpox ranges from 10 to 21 days, but is usually 14 to 15 days. In contrast to the localised lesions of herpes zoster, chickenpox lesions are scattered. In otherwise healthy children, secondary skin and soft-tissue infections are the commonest complications of chickenpox, and are found in 1–4% of cases, accounting for more than half of the chickenpox hospital admissions; *Staphylococcus aureus* and group A beta-haemolytic streptococci are commonly involved (Tarlow and Walters, 1998). Chickenpox in adults is more severe than in children, with a wider range of complications, especially varicella pneumonitis. Occupational and infection control aspects of varicella have been recently reviewed (Burns et al, 1998).

Aciclovir is the only currently available treatment for chickenpox in the UK. If VZ immunoglobulin is given to susceptible, high-risk contacts early in the incubation period, chickenpox can be attenuated or prevented. A live, attenuated varicella vaccine is currently available in the UK only on a named-patient basis for immunocompromised individuals (Ogilvie, 1998).

Cytomegalovirus (CMV) disease during pregnancy is discussed in Chapter 10. The main features of CMV inclusion disease of the newborn include jaundice, hepatosplenomegaly and microcephaly, often with long-term neurological sequelae such as mental retardation and sensorineural deafness. The major skin manifestations are petechiae and blueberry-muffin type lesions. Although blueberry-muffin babies were commonly seen following congenital rubella, they are now almost exclusively seen with CMV (Krafchik, 1996).

Epstein-Barr virus (EBV) causes glandular fever, or infectious mononucleosis. Almost all patients with glandular fever who are treated with ampicillin develop a maculopapular rash (Fig 7.8). The Gianotti-Crosti syndrome (acral papular dermatitis of childhood) occurs in young children who remain well, while pink papules develop on the face and extremities. Lymphadenopathy and hepatosplenomegaly may occur, and the eruption disappears after four to six weeks with no sequelae. The syndrome is associated with infection with different viruses, but EBV is a common cause in the United States (Krafchik, 1996).

In 1986, human herpesvirus type 6 (HHV-6) was discovered as a result of research into AIDS and lymphoproliferative diseases. There are at least two types of HHV-6: HHV-6A and HHV-6B (Braun et al, 1997). In 1988

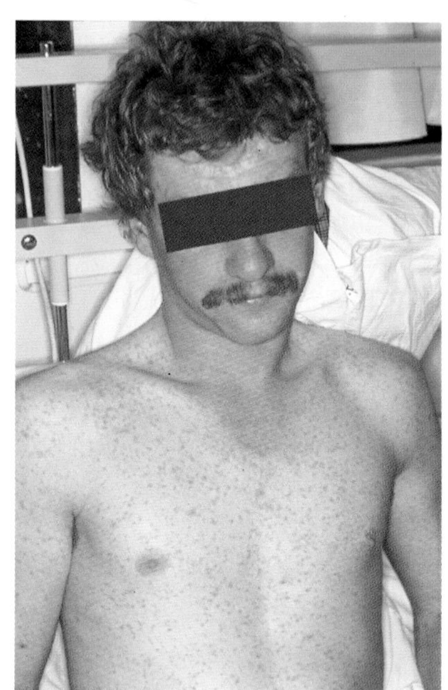

Fig 7.8 Ampicillin rash, following treatment for glandular fever
Source: Courtesy of Dr Sheila M. Burns, Regional Clinical Virology Laboratory, City Hospital, Edinburgh EH10 5SB

HHV-6B was found to be the cause of exanthem subitum (roseola infantum or sixth disease), which usually occurs as a primary infection between infancy and three years of age, probably after transfer via saliva from mother to infant. Usually, after the high fever which lasts three to five days has settled, a macular or maculopapular rash develops, beginning on the trunk and often spreading to the face and neck. However, recent studies have shown that many primary HHV-6 infections do not have this classical presentation (Braun et al, 1997); for example, vesicular lesions occurred in one case.

Primary infection with human herpesvirus type 7 (HHV-7) has occasionally been associated with exanthem subitum, and other rashes similar to measles and rubella (Braun et al, 1997). The recently described association of HHV-7 with pityriasis rosea has stimulated debate on the role of certain herpesviruses in the reactivation of other herpesviruses, and whether single agents are exclusively responsible for particular infectious diseases (Drago et al, 1998).

Kaposi's sarcoma (KS) is the commonest neoplasm seen in AIDS patients, and is found in a high proportion of HIV-infected male homosexuals (Fig 7.9), although it is rare in HIV-infected children. KS can also be found in a small proportion of immunosuppressed patients following transplantation, and in non-HIV-infected Africans in HIV-endemic areas of Africa (Offerman, 1996). Human herpesvirus type 8 (HHV-8) has been found in KS lesions from all risk groups worldwide. However, in the United States' general population, about 25% of adults (including volunteer blood donors) and 2–8% of children have been infected with HHV-8 (Lennette et al, 1996). It seems that HHV-8 infection is associated primarily with sexual transmission, but there may also be a non-sexual route.

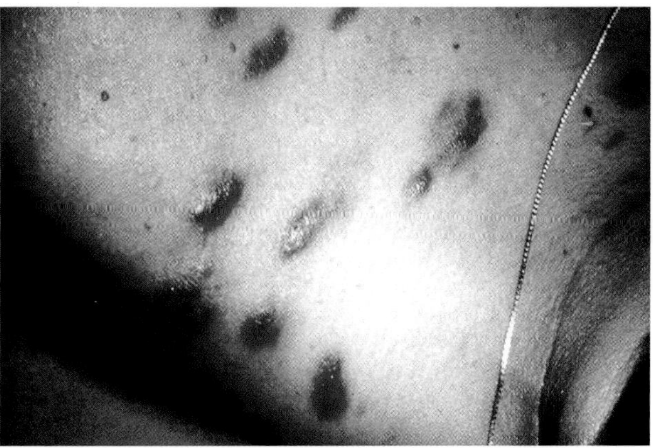

Fig 7.9 Kaposi's sarcoma
Source: Courtesy of Dr Sheila M. Burns, Regional Clinical Virology Laboratory, City Hospital, Edinburgh EH10 5SB

Parvovirus B19

Human parvovirus B19, a small, single-stranded DNA virus, is a common infectious agent. Infection may be asymptomatic or may cause erythema infectiosum in children, post-infection arthropathy in adults, bone-marrow failure in immunosuppressed patients and aplastic crisis in patients with diminished red cell survival. When a foetus becomes infected with B19, hydrops foetalis and death may result (Kerr and Umene, 1997).

B19 is a common infection of humans, occurring both sporadically and in outbreaks. In the UK B19 infection usually occurs in an epidemic cycle of two high-incidence years followed by two low-incidence years (*CDR Weekly*, 1998).

A distinguishing feature of erythema infectiosum is the classic 'slapped cheek' appearance that precedes a maculopapular eruption in the proximal extremities, giving a characteristic lacy pattern (Krafchik, 1996). This is due to deposits of immune complexes, formed as a result of the vigorous immune response stimulated in children by large numbers of viruses released directly into the bloodstream from lysed erythroblastoid precursor cells.

Papillomaviruses

In humans warts are caused by human papillomaviruses (HPV), of which there are at least 83 types. Viral warts are rare under five years of age, and most common between 12 and 16 years, with successful transmission dependent on inoculation through a breach in the surface of the skin or mucosa (Bunney et al, 1992).

There are cutaneous, or skin, warts and mucocutaneous warts. Skin warts can be divided into three groups:

- deep plantar warts, or verrucas
- common warts
- plane warts

The eventual disappearance of skin warts largely depends on a good cell-mediated immune response. However, HPVs can pose major problems in patients with deficient cell-mediated immunity.

Mucocutaneous warts affect the urogenital, anorectal and upper respiratory areas. Genital warts are the commonest sexually transmitted viral infection in the UK, and accounted for 22% of all diagnoses made in genitourinary medicine clinics in England in 1996 (Simms et al, 1998). With mounting evidence which implicates certain types of HPV in cervical and other lower genital cancers, the possible role of HPV screening in the diagnosis of cervical disease and the prospects of a HPV vaccine are presently being evaluated (McCance, 1998).

Measles

The availability of an effective vaccine means that measles is no longer an unavoidable childhood disease. Nevertheless, although a relatively benign disease in healthy children, measles is one of the commonest causes of infant mortality in Third World countries with poor standards of nutrition. For example, worldwide, measles accounts for about one million deaths annually among children under five years of age (Centers for Disease Control and Prevention, 1998).

Measles infects through the upper respiratory tract or conjunctiva. About 14 days later the characteristic maculopapular rash begins behind the ears and on the forehead, spreading over the body, and fading three to four days later. The rash is preceded by the pathognomonic Koplik's spots, which appear in the mouth, opposite the lower molars. Otitis media is the commonest complication of measles. Giant-cell pneumonia may occur as a complication in immunocompromised children and is often fatal. The main neurological sequelae of measles are acute post-infectious measles encephalomyelitis, measles inclusion body encephalitis, and the rare subacute sclerosing panencephalitis.

Following the eradication of smallpox, and the near-elimination of poliomyelitis, the global elimination of measles is feasible, and it is hoped that measles might be eliminated from the World Health Organisation European Region by 2007 (Centers for Disease Control and Prevention, 1998).

In the UK, measles is declining. For instance, in the late 1980s, between 50,000 and 100,000 cases of measles were notified annually to the Office for National Statistics (ONS), as it now is: in 1995, only 7,768 cases of measles were notified to the ONS (Gay et al, 1997).

Other viruses

Since vaccination against measles, mumps and rubella was introduced in the UK in 1988, the incidence of these diseases has fallen to low levels. In view of adverse publicity about the measles, mumps and rubella (MMR) vaccine, it is worth noting that the Medical Research Council's expert group met in 1998 and found no evidence of an association between either measles or MMR vaccine and autism or bowel disease (Chief Medical Officer, 1998).

Unlike measles, the rubella rash varies in appearance, if it appears at all. A clinical diagnosis of rubella is unreliable and laboratory tests are essential, especially given the implications of rubella infection in pregnancy. Immunisation has been successful in reducing the risk of transmission of rubella to pregnant women in developed countries. It now appears that more young men than women are susceptible to rubella (Miller et al, 1997).

The skin can be a target organ for many enteroviruses, yet – with exceptions such as Coxsackie virus type A16 – rashes are uncommon, but may be morbilliform, rubelliform, vesicular and petechial in nature.

Other virus infections involving the skin include viral haemorrhagic fevers such as Lassa fever, Marburg disease and dengue. However, the rashes associated with these diseases are not sufficiently distinctive to be pathognomonic.

References

Arvin, A. M. (1996) Varicella-zoster virus. *Clinical Microbiology Reviews*; 9: 3, 361–381.

Birthistle, K., Carrington, D. (1997) Molluscum contagiosum virus. *Journal of Infection*; 34: 21–28.

Braun, D. K., Dominguez, G., Pellett, P. E. (1997) Human herpesvirus 6. *Clinical Microbiology Reviews*; 10: 3, 521–567.

Bunney, M. H., Benton, C., Cubie, H. A. (1992) The epidemiology, infectivity, transmission, and prevention of warts. In: *Viral Warts, Biology and Treatment*. Oxford: Oxford University Press, 2nd edn.

Burns, S. M., Mitchell-Heggs, N., Carrington, D. (1998) Occupational and infection control aspects of varicella. *Journal of Infection*; 36: suppl. 1, 73–78.

Carrington, D. (1996) Treating genital herpes. *British Journal of Sexual Medicine*; March/April, 14–17.

CDR Weekly (1998) Rising incidence of parvovirus B19 infection; 8: 11, 93.

Centers for Disease Control and Prevention (1998) Advances in global measles control and elimination: summary of the 1997 international meeting. *Morbidity and Mortality Weekly Report*; 47: no. RR-11, 1–23.

Chief Medical Officer *Measles, MMR Vaccine, Crohn's Disease and Autism*. London: Department of Health (PL/CMO/92/2).

Drago, F., Ranieri, E., Rebora, A. (1998) Pityriasis rosea and herpesvirus 7: action or interaction? *Dermatology*; 197: 275.

Ellner, P. D. (1998) Smallpox: gone but not forgotten. *Infection*; 26: 5, 263–9.

Gay, N., Ramsay, M., Cohen, B. et al (1997). The epidemiology of measles in England and Wales since the 1994 vaccination campaign. *CDR Review*; 7: 2, R17–R21.

Kerr, J. R., Umene, K. (1997) The molecular epidemiology of parvovirus B19. *Reviews in Medical Microbiology*; 8: 1, 21–31.

Krafchik, B. R. (1996) Advances in viral infections. *Advances in Dermatology*; 11: 155–177.

Lennette, E. T., Blackbourn, D. J., Levy, J. A. (1996) Antibodies to human herpesvirus type 8 in the general population and in Kaposi's sarcoma patients. *Lancet*; 348: 858–861.

McCance, D. J. (1998) Human papillomaviruses and cervical cancer. *Journal of Medical Microbiology*; 47: 371–373.

Miller, E., Waight, P., Gay, N. et al (1997) The epidemiology of rubella in England and Wales before and after the 1994 measles and rubella vaccination campaign: fourth joint report from the PHLS and the National Congenital Rubella Surveillance Programme. *CDR Review*; 7: 2, R26–R32.

Monath, T. P. (1995) Dengue: the risk to developed and developing countries. In: Roizman, B. (ed.) *Infectious Diseases in an Age of Change*, Washington, DC: National Academy of Sciences.

Noble, W. C. (1981) *Microbiology of Human Skin*. London: Lloyd-Luke (Medical Books).

Offerman, M. K. (1996) HHV-8: a new herpesvirus associated with Kaposi's sarcoma. *Trends in Microbiology*; 4: 10, 383–385.

Ogilvie, M. M. (1998) Antiviral prophylaxis and treatment in chickenpox. *Journal of Infection*; 36: suppl. 1, 31–38.

Postlethwaite, R. (1970) Molluscum contagiosum — a review. *Archives of Environmental Health*; 21: 432–452.

Robinson, T. W. E., Heath, R. B. (1983a) Smallpox and other poxvirus infections of man. In: *Virus Diseases and the Skin*. Edinburgh: Churchill Livingstone.

Robinson, T. W. E., Heath, R. B. (1983b) Infections with herpes simplex virus. In: *Virus Diseases and the Skin*. Edinburgh: Churchill Livingstone.

Simms, I., Hughes, G., Swan, A. V. et al (1998) New cases seen at genitourinary medicine clinics: England 1996. *CDR Supplement*; 8: suppl. 1, S1–S11.

Tarlow, M. J., Walters, S. (1998) Chickenpox in childhood. *Journal of Infection*; 36: suppl. 1, 39–47.

WHO Meeting (1985) Prevention and control of herpesvirus diseases. Part 2: Epidemiology and immunology. *Bulletin of the World Health Organisation;* 63: 3, 427–444.

8 The central nervous system

When God endowed human beings with brains, He did not intend to guarantee them.

Baron de Montesquieu (1689–1755).

Neurovirology studies the effects of viruses and other transmissible agents on the nervous system. It began with Louis Pasteur's work on rabies, which culminated in the first rabies vaccine in 1885, and now reaches beyond the virological spectrum to embrace prions, and includes the recently recognised new variant Creutzfeldt-Jacob disease (nvCJD).

Viruses may invade the central nervous system (CNS) by different routes. When large numbers of viruses are circulating in the blood, the cerebrospinal fluid (CSF) can be reached by leakage across blood capillaries in the meninges or choroid plexus. For example, enteroviruses and the viruses of lymphocytic choriomeningitis and mumps, which cause aseptic meningitis in man, reach the CSF by this means. In contrast, rabies virus favours a more direct approach, where peripheral nerves may be breached by the bite of a an infected dog, for instance, whence the virus slowly progresses to the CNS.

Viral encephalitis can be classified as:

- acute encephalitis
- acute post-infectious encephalomyelitis
- chronic viral encephalopathies

In acute encephalitis, neurons are damaged as a direct result of viral replication, there is an acute inflammatory response, and demyelination is absent. It can be either epidemic or sporadic. Epidemic disease includes that caused by arboviruses and enteroviruses, whereas sporadic viral encephalitis may be caused by herpes simplex virus (HSV), varicella zoster virus (VZV), cytomegalovirus (CMV), mumps virus, measles virus and rabies virus.

Symptoms of acute post-infectious encephalomyelitis usually begin 10 to 14 days after infection of other organs by viruses such as VZV, CMV and measles virus. It seems that the viral infection sets off an immunological reaction, with widespread demyelination.

The chronic viral encephalopathies consist of those involving an inflammatory reaction in the brain, such as subacute sclerosing panencephalitis (SSPE) and progressive multifocal leucoencephalopathy (PML), and congenital encephalopathies following *in utero* infection of the foetus by, for example, rubella and CMV. Twenty years ago this group would have included the agent of Creutzfeldt-Jakob disease (CJD) and bovine spongiform encephalopathy (BSE). However, these transmissible spongiform encephalopathies are strongly associated with the prion agents, and are now classified separately.

HERPESVIRUSES

Herpes simplex virus

Meningitis and encephalitis are the most frequent and important CNS complications of herpes simplex virus (HSV) infection. Although many cases of primary genital herpes are due to HSV type 1 (HSV-1), most cases of meningitis associated with primary genital herpes are caused by HSV type 2 (HSV-2).

HSV encephalitis can occur during the neonatal and post-neonatal period. Although both HSV types can cause neonatal HSV encephalitis, HSV-1 is thought to produce less severe disease.

HSV is probably the commonest cause of sporadic viral encephalitis, with the majority outside the neonatal period thought to be caused by HSV-1: the results of a recent study of 64 cases (Dennett et al, 1997) suggest that in the UK, only about 2% of cases of HSV encephalitis are caused by HSV-2. Men and women can be affected at any age, with no apparent seasonal or geographical distribution. It is unclear whether HSV encephalitis is the result of primary infection, reinfection or reactivation of latent infection (Klapper and Cleator, 1997). What is clear is that the condition is serious and life-threatening, with frequent neurological sequelae and deficit.

Varicella zoster virus

Primary infection by, and recurrence of, VZV can produce CNS infection and disease. The main neurological complications of varicella are of the 'post-infectious' type, caused by an abnormal immune response. Thus acute disseminated encephalomyelitis is an acute 'post-infectious' demyelinating disease that may lead to acute cerebellar ataxia, which is the commonest neurological complication associated with varicella infection. Encephalitis is a less common, but more severe complication of varicella, affecting 0.1–0.2% of patients (Echevarria et al, 1997).

In contrast to acute VZV infection, neurological syndromes associated with recurrences are often the result of viral replication in the CNS, which is reached via the bloodstream or by direct spread from sensory ganglia, where it remains latent. Post-herpetic neuralgia is the commonest neurological complication of herpes zoster, affecting 7–35% of patients. In addition, acute encephalitis, aseptic meningitis and myelitis are also neurological complications of herpes zoster, with and without the presence of a cutaneous rash (Echevarria et al, 1997).

Cytomegalovirus

Human cytomegalovirus (CMV) is a common virus which does not usually cause symptomatic disease in immunocompetent individuals. However, the consequences of CMV infection are most devastating in congenitally infected infants and immunosuppressed patients, including those with AIDS, with CMV infections of the CNS occurring in both groups. In cytomegalic inclusion disease, the severest form of congenital CMV infection, the brain is the main target organ, with manifestations including microcephaly, paralysis, seizures, mental retardation and deafness. Whereas CMV infection of the CNS has been described in up to one-third of AIDS autopsy cases (Cinque et al, 1997), only 12% of 573 reported cases of CMV encephalitis occurred in immunocompromised non-AIDS patients (Arribas et al, 1996). The two main manifestations of CMV encephalitis in AIDS patients are ventriculoencephalitis and micronodular encephalitis (Cinque et al, 1997).

Laboratory diagnosis and treatment

Herpesviruses cannot be easily cultured from CSF. Nevertheless, the polymerase chain reaction (PCR) has proved a valuable aid to early diagnosis of herpesvirus CNS infections by detecting the presence of viral deoxyribonucleic acid (DNA) in the CSF. However, it is largely confined to specialist centres, and quality assurance is an important consideration in the application of this highly sensitive technique.

Aciclovir is the only antiviral agent currently available for the treatment of HSV infection of the CNS, and aciclovir is the treatment of choice for VZV infections. In both cases early treatment is essential to be effective.

Ganciclovir and foscarnet are currently used for the treatment of CMV CNS infections, with cidofovir a recent addition. However, the current antiviral treatments for CMV can be problematic. For example, myelotoxicity with the use of ganciclovir has limited its use in the treatment of both adults and congenitally infected infants, and the development of ganciclovir-resistant strains of CMV may explain the failure of ganciclovir treatment in AIDS patients with encephalitis.

ENTEROVIRUSES

Although there are 66 types of enterovirus known to infect humans, several types have been reclassified over the years, which explains why some types have numbers greater than 66. Most enterovirus infections are asymptomatic, but the main CNS manifestations of enterovirus infection are paralytic poliomyelitis, aseptic meningitis and encephalitis.

Paralytic poliomyelitis is caused by poliovirus, of which there are three serotypes. The main feature of the disease is acute flaccid paralysis as a result of lower motor neuron damage. The success of vaccination, which began in 1955, has resulted in the virtual eradication of poliomyelitis. However, a similar paralytic illness has been associated with Coxsackie virus type A7, and enterovirus types 70 and 71.

The main clinical features of aseptic meningitis are headache, photophobia, neck stiffness, fever and nausea, with clinical recovery often occurring within one week (Muir and van Loon, 1997). Most enteroviruses, including poliovirus, have been associated with aseptic meningitis. It is important to distinguish viral meningitis from the more serious bacterial meningitis if appropriate antibiotic therapy is to begin.

Blood glucose and CSF protein concentrations, and the number of polymorphonuclear lymphocytes in blood and CSF, are usually lower in aseptic meningitis than bacterial meningitis. The recent introduction of PCR for the detection of enteroviruses in CSF should help in the management of patients with meningitis. Establishing a viral cause could avoid unnecessary antibiotic treatment and laboratory tests, and hasten hospital discharge (Muir and van Loon, 1997). With the exception of poliovirus, enteroviruses are easily recovered from CSF during the acute phase of aseptic meningitis.

Encephalitis is an unusual outcome of enterovirus infection, and cases often have symptoms of both meningitis and encephalitis (meningoencephalitis), with potentially fatal consequences (Zuckerman et al, 1993). Because of currently available rapid diagnostic molecular techniques, brain biopsy is rarely used in the diagnosis of viral encephalitis.

Arboviruses

These viruses are transmitted from one vertebrate host to another by bloodsucking arthropods, inside which they multiply without evidence of disease or damage. The most efficient vectors of arboviruses are mosquitoes, ticks, sandflies and biting midges. Clearly, the geographical distribution of arbovirus diseases will be determined to a large extent by the ecology of the relevant arthropods. In terms of the natural history of arboviruses, man is an incidental host who becomes infected after a chance encounter with an arthropod in which the virus occurs naturally, or which has acquired virus from a cycle involving birds or wild or domesticated animals.

The arboviruses belong to three different viral families, *Togaviridae, Flaviviridae* and *Bunyaviridae.* More than 100 arboviruses can infect humans without necessarily causing overt disease. In the UK louping ill virus, carried by the tick *Ixodes ricinus,* is the only indigenous arbovirus and causes few human infections. The possibility of an arbovirus infection should be considered in patients who develop unexplained fevers within a fortnight after arrival in the UK from arbovirus endemic regions abroad.

Arbovirus infections in humans may produce three types of clinical syndromes:

- fevers, with or without a maculopapular rash
- haemorrhagic fevers, often severe and fatal
- encephalitis, often with a high case-fatality rate

In an arbovirus epidemic it is probable that less than 1% of those infected will have detectable clinical CNS signs; the majority have no detectable illness (Webb, 1975). In the United States, during 1996–97, 252 cases of La Crosse encephalitis occurred, with one fatality; 19 cases of eastern equine encephalitis occurred, with five fatalaties; and 15 cases of St Louis encephalitis occurred, with two fatalaties (US Department of Health, 1998).

Rabies

Although no cases of human rabies have been acquired in the UK since 1902, 12 people since then have died from rabies in the UK; all had been infected abroad. With some urging a change in the present UK Quarantine Regulations, others have reappraised the risks of importing rabies into the country and found the existing regulations do not cover all of the risks posed by the disease (Scott, 1998). For example, some dogs that have recovered from rabies can become rabies carriers, and occasionally shed virus in their saliva. Clearly, rabies represents an ever-present threat.

The commonest mode of infection is by the bite of a rabid animal, and infected domestic dogs pose the greatest threat to humans in urban environments. The incubation period may range from four days to 19 years, but is typically between 30 and 90 days. Following entry into the peripheral nerves, rabies virus moves towards the spinal cord and brain at a rough speed of 3mm per hour (Nicholson, 1987). After viral replication in the CNS, the virus moves back along nerve routes to salivary glands and other tissues, where more virus multiplication occurs. Recovery from clinical rabies is rare, although the disease may be avoided if post-exposure vaccine treatment is instituted as soon as possible.

However, a bite from a rabid animal does not necessarily cause disease. Indeed, rabies virus seems to be able to induce atypical inapparent infections in humans. For example, in a survey of Nigerian dog owners, 100 out of 350 owners had rabies antibodies in their serum (Ogunkoya: cited in Scott, 1998).

Measles

With measles now a candidate for possible global eradication, vaccination programmes have achieved a huge decrease in the incidence of acute measles in the developed world, yet measles and its complications remain a serious public health problem in developing countries.

The three main CNS complications of measles virus infections are:

- acute post-infectious measles encephalomyelitis (APME)
- measles inclusion body encephalitis (MIBE)
- subacute sclerosing panencephalitis (SSPE)

APME has an incidence of one in 1,000 cases of measles, usually occurring within a fortnight after onset of the rash; measles virus cannot be isolated from brain tissue in cases of APME; it is thought to be caused by an autoimmune response (Liebert, 1997).

MIBE and SSPE are the result of a persistent measles virus infection of the CNS, with MIBE occurring as an opportunistic infection among immunocompromised patients, following a progressive course within weeks to months after measles.

First seen in Belfast in 1965 (Bellman and Dick, 1978), SSPE is a chronic progressive inflammatory CNS disease with a fatal outcome. With an incidence of about one per million of the childhood population of the UK, and seen more often in males, the mean age at onset was 9.8 years, and it was estimated that the risk of SSPE following natural measles is about five to 20 times higher than that following measles vaccination (Bellman and Dick, 1978). As expected, those countries whose vaccination programmes have seen a decline in the incidence of acute measles, have also seen a concomitant decrease in measles complications including SSPE.

Polyomavirus

JC virus is a polyomavirus which causes PML, a disease of immunosuppressed patients, and the only human demyelinating disease known to be caused by a virus. Although more than 80% of the adult population are infected with JC virus, only a small minority of immunosuppressed patients develop the disease (Weber, 1997). However, with the advent of AIDS, the incidence of PML has greatly increased, and it affects 2–4% of individuals with advanced human immunodeficiency virus (HIV) disease (Fong and Toma, 1995). Mono- and/or hemiparesis is the commonest neurological presenting sign, and magnetic resonance imaging is the diagnostic tool of choice for investigating suspected PML.

Transmissible spongiform encephalopathies

The group of fatal dementias associated with post-mortem spongiform changes in the brain are called transmissible spongiform encephalopathies (TSEs), and their importance has increased since the outbreak of bovine spongiform encephalopathy (BSE) in the UK, and the cases of new variant Creutzfeldt-Jakob disease (nvCJD) that are thought to have occurred as a result.

In the 1920s Creutzfeldt and Jakob independently described a fatal neurological disorder. CJD is related to other rare transmissible neurological disorders, including:

- kuru, spread by ritualistic cannibalism (a now defunct custom) among the Fore tribe of New Guinea
- the Gerstmann-Straussler-Scheinker syndrome, a rare inherited form of progressive cerebellar ataxia
- fatal familial insomnia, another inherited condition
- scrapie, an endemic disease of sheep and goats in the UK and other European countries (Ironside, 1998)

The agents of these diseases are resistant to the physical and chemical treatments which would inactivate conventional viruses and bacteria, and are widely considered to be prions. It is thought that a normal cell-surface glycoprotein, called a prion protein, is somehow caused to undergo a conformational change. It is this altered protein which accumulates in the brain in CJD and related disorders.

In 1986 BSE was identified in cattle in the UK (Table 8.1), and in 1990 the CJD Surveillance Unit began monitoring cases of CJD. By 1996 10 young adults had succumbed to a new variant of CJD, and subsequent transmission experiments using monkeys and mice indicated that the BSE agent was the cause (Ironside, 1998).

1985	(Apr)	BSE first observed clinically
1986	(Nov)	Disease identified as spongiform encephalopathy
1987	(Apr)	Initial epidemiological studies started
1987	(Dec)	Initial epidemiological studies incriminate ruminant-derived MBM as a cause of BSE
1988	(Apr)	Southwood Committee set up
	(July)	Ruminant feed ban introduced for MBM
	(Aug)	All cattle with symptoms of BSE to be slaughtered
1989	(Feb)	Southwood report; risk to humans 'remote'; estimates expected number of cattle with BSE to reach 17,000–25,000
	(Nov)	Ban on use of certain bovine offals for human consumption
1991	(Mar)	EU bans export of British cattle over 6 months old
	(Apr)	EU bans export of British offal
	(May)	First case of 'BSE' in cat
	(Sept)	Offal banned from animal feed
1992		BSE epidemic peaks at 36,681 cases in a year
1993	(July)	100,000th confirmed case of BSE
1994	(Nov)	Thymus and intestines added to offal ban; all mammalian protein banned from cattle and sheep feed
1995	(Nov)	First 3 deaths of younger humans
1996	(Mar)	Suspected link between BSE and nvCJD; EU bans all British beef exports
	(July)	Controls on slaughter of sheep
1997	(Dec)	Ban on sale of beef on the bone because of infectivity in spinal cord and possibly in bone marrow

Table 8.1 The chronology of the BSE epidemic
Source: Reprinted from P. N. Campbell (1998)
Reproduced with permission of S. Karger AG, Basle

Opinion is divided on the nature of the threat which nvCJD poses to the public. For example, while some suggest that intraspecies transfer of the disease is likely through blood transfusion (Lacey, 1998), others consider it a more remote possibility (Turner and Ironside, 1998). In December 1997 the sale of beef on the bone was banned because of a perceived risk of infectivity in the spinal cord and, possibly, the bone marrow (Campbell, 1998). A recent report considers the fact that the average person runs a one-in-one-thousand-million risk of getting nvCJD from T-bone steak in a year, and defines an epidemiologist 'as someone who eats T-bone steaks but doesn't bet on the Lottery' (*SCIEH Weekly Report*, 1998).

References

Arribas, J. R., Storch, G. A., Clifford, D. B., Tselis, A. C. (1996) Cytomegalovirus encephalitis. *Annals of Internal Medicine*; 125: 577–587.

Bellman, M. H., Dick, G. W. A. (1978) Surveillance of subacute sclerosing panencephalitis. *Journal of the Royal College of Physicians*; 12: 3, 256–261.

Campbell, P. N. (1998) Bovine spongiform encephalopathy (BSE) – mad cow disease. *Medical Principles and Practice*; 7: 172–186.

Cinque, P., Marenzi, R., Ceresa, D. (1997) Cytomegalovirus infections of the nervous system. *Intervirology*; 40: 85–97.

Dennett, C., Cleator, G. M., Klapper, P. E. (1997) HSV-1 and HSV-2 in herpes simplex encephalitis: a study of sixty-four cases in the United Kingdom. *Journal of Medical Virology*; 53: 1–3.

Echevarria, J. M., Casas, I., Martinez-Martin, P. (1997) Infections of the nervous system caused by varicella-zoster virus: a review. *Intervirology*; 40: 72–84.

Fong, I. W., Toma, E. (1995) The natural history of progressive multifocal leucoencephalopathy in patients with AIDS. *Clinical Infectious Diseases*; 20: 1305–1310.

Ironside, J. W. (1998) Creutzfeldt-Jakob disease – the story so far. *Proceedings of the Royal College of Physicians of Edinburgh*; 28: 143–149.

Klapper, P. E., Cleator, G. M. (1997) Herpes simplex virus. *Intervirology*; 40: 62–71.

Lacey, R. (1998) Bovine spongiform encephalopathy: the fall-out. *Reviews in Medical Microbiology*; 9: 3, 119–127.

Liebert, U. G. (1997) Measles virus infections of the central nervous system. *Intervirology*; 40: 176–184.

Muir, P., Van Loon, A. M. (1997) Enterovirus infections of the central nervous system. *Intervirology*; 40: 153–166.

Nicholson, K. G. (1987) Rabies. In: Zuckerman, A. J., Banatvala, J. E., Pattison, J. R. (eds) *Principles and Practice of Clinical Virology*, Chichester: John Wiley & Sons.

SCIEH Weekly Report (1998) When is a CJD risk a risk and what does it actually mean?; 32: 98/08, 45.

Scott, G. R. (1998) Rabies: false, forgotten and fresh findings. *Proceedings of the Royal College of Physicians of Edinburgh*; 28: 198–206.

Turner, M. L., Ironside, J. W. (1998) New-variant Creutzfeldt-Jakob disease: the risk of transmission by blood transfusion. *Blood Reviews*; 12: 255–268.

US Department of Health and Human Services (1998) Arboviral infections of the central nervous system – United States, 1996–1997. *Morbidity and Mortality Weekly Report*; 47: 25, 517–522.

Webb, H. E. (1975) The arbovirus encephalitides. In: Illis, L. S. (ed.) *Viral Diseases of the Central Nervous System*. London: Baillière Tindall.

Weber, T. (1997) Editorial. *Intervirology*; 40: 59–61.

Zuckerman, M. A., Sheaff, M., Martin, J. E., Gabriel, C. M. (1993) Fatal case of echovirus type 9 encephalitis. *Journal of Clinical Pathology*; 46: 865–866.

9 The eye

By heaven, the wonder in a mortal eye!

William Shakespeare (1564–1616), *Love's Labour's Lost.*

Viruses infect us either through mucous membranes or the skin. The mucous membranes line the respiratory tract, the gastrointestinal tract, the genital tract and the conjunctiva. Infection through the mucous membranes is less traumatic than infection through the skin, and epithelial cells are directly available for infecting viruses to attach themselves to. However, those viruses settling on the conjunctiva are not given free ingress by the host. The conjunctiva is gently washed with tears, protective secretions containing anti-microbial agents such as lysozyme, which is particularly effective against certain bacteria. In the blinking of an eye, the moist surface of the conjunctiva is swept by the eyelid, clearing away dust, grime and microbes, which are dumped in the nasal cavity by way of the tear ducts.

The best chance for a virus is to take advantage of any breaches that might occur in this natural defence: for example, disease affecting the cleansing and/or blinking mechanisms, minor injuries by foreign bodies, or direct mechanical infection by fingers and insects. Bathing provides ample opportunity for microbes to splash onto the conjunctiva, and eyes may become irritated in chemically treated swimming pools. The conjunctiva has a special relationship with the genital tract, in that both seem to be equally favoured by many sexually transmissible infections, most of which can affect the eye to varying degrees (Gillies and Donovan, 1998). As well as being susceptible to direct infection from the outside, the conjunctiva can also be infected from the inside, as occurs during acute episodes of measles.

In our consideration of viral infections of the eye, it is appropriate to include chlamydia. Chlamydia are bacteria, but their level of complexity falls between viruses and bacteria. For example, chlamydia cannot be grown on an agar plate like most other bacteria; they replicate only inside living cells, yet they are susceptible to antibiotic treatment. Historically, the laboratory diagnosis of chlamydial infection has been chiefly undertaken in virus laboratories, making chlamydia 'honorary viruses', as it were.

Herpes simplex virus (HSV) and adenovirus are the two viruses most likely to spring to mind when thinking of viral infections of the eye. However, there are members of at least 14 different virus families which cause disease, with infection of the epithelium of the cornea, conjunctiva and eyelid the most common clinical manifestation. On rare occasions Creutzfeldt-Jakob disease (caused by a prion, not a virus) and rabies have been transmitted by infected corneal grafts (Darrell, 1985a).

Chlamydia

There are four members of the genus *Chlamydia*: *C. trachomatis, C. pneumoniae, C. psittaci* and *C. pecorum*. *C. trachomatis* causes three distinct syndromes:

- lymphogranuloma venereum, a sexually transmitted disease especially prevalent in the tropics and subtropics
- oculogenital infections
- trachoma

Trachoma is an ancient disease, referred to by Hippocrates and Galen, and described in the Egyptian Ebers papyrus, written about 3,800 years ago. It is mainly endemic in tropical and subtropical countries, especially North Africa, the Middle East and northern India, where it is associated with poor standards of hygiene. The most common infectious cause of blindness, trachoma affects at least 400 million people worldwide, with 20 million blinded by it. It is a keratoconjunctivitis, spread from eye to eye, and is especially associated with serotypes A, B, Ba and C (Schachter et al, 1998).

C. trachomatis, serotypes D–K, causes a sexually transmitted disease that may also produce inclusion conjunctivitis. In contrast to trachoma, which is spread by eye to eye, adult inclusion conjunctivitis is mainly a sexually transmitted disease, acquired by autoinoculation, or direct or indirect contact with the genital secretions of an infected person. The lower eyelid is more affected than the upper eyelid in inclusion conjunctivitis, whereas the converse applies in trachoma.

Conjunctivitis with discharge occurring in the first month of life is referred to as ophthalmia neonatorum, the commonest bacterial cause being *C. trachomatis*. Around one baby in three exposed to the organism in the birth canal will develop the disease (Gillies and Donovan, 1998).

Traditionally, the laboratory diagnosis of chlamydial infection relied on the detection of the organism in cell cultures. This is expensive, time-consuming, and is not routinely used. Direct antigen techniques such as immunofluorescence and enzyme immunoassay are less complicated than cell culture, and give quicker results. However, refinements in nucleic acid amplification technology continue, and the ligase chain reaction (LCR) is an increasingly favoured diagnostic test that offers a quick, highly sensitive, nonculture method for detecting *C. trachomatis* (McCartney et al, 1998).

Herpesviruses

Of the eight human herpesviruses, six have been associated with eye infections.

HSV is one of the commonest causes of corneal blindness in the world, with around 500,000 cases of HSV eye infection in the United States, annually (Darougar et al, 1985). Although HSV types 1 and 2 can each cause eye and genital disease, HSV infections of the eye are usually caused by HSV-1, except in neonates where HSV-2 is the main cause. There are two clinical types: primary and recurrent. Primary infection occurs mainly in children, where it is generally asymptomatic, although there may be mild to severe conjunctivitis and corneal ulceration. It is a self-limiting disease, but recurs in around 25% of patients. In recurrent infection, the cornea is chiefly affected, with usually only one eye involved.

During chickenpox, although vesicles appear on the eyelids and conjunctivae, eye complications are rare. However, varicella dendritic keratitis has been documented as a complication of chickenpox (Uchida, 1985), and in the rare congenital varicella syndrome, chorioretinitis, microphthalmia and cataracts can occur (Arvin, 1996). Herpes zoster occurs mainly in older adults, varying in severity from mild to severe, with the ophthalmic division of the trigeminal nerve being affected in around 7% of cases. Ocular manifestations of ophthalmic zoster include conjunctivitis, acute keratitis and iritis. Ocular complications of zoster tend to recur, from one month to 10 years after the initial episode (Marsh, 1985). Between 5% and 15% of human immunodeficiency virus- (HIV-) positive patients are affected by herpes zoster ophthalmicus (Jabs and Quinn, cited in Cunningham and Margolis, 1998).

Until the 1970s there were few reports of cytomegalovirus (CMV) eye infections in adults. The rise in the number of transplant recipients has led to more iatrogenically immunosuppressed patients. This, together with the immunosuppression associated with the advent of the acquired immunodeficiency syndrome (AIDS) has seen an increase in CMV-associated eye infections, the main feature of which is chorioretinitis (Fig 9.1). Whereas CMV retinitis can affect between 30% and 40% of HIV-positive patients (Ives, 1997), it occurs infrequently in transplant patients, usually presenting more than six months after transplantation (LaRocco and Burgert, 1997).

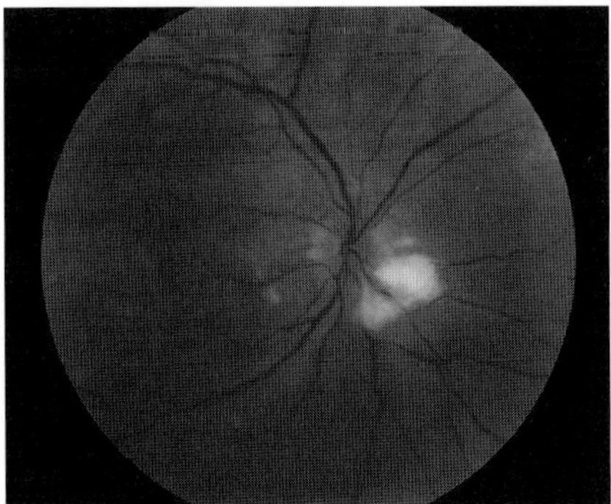

Fig 9.1 CMV retinitis
Source: Courtesy of Dr Sheila M. Burns, Regional Clinical Virology Laboratory, City Hospital, Edinburgh EH10 5SB

In 1973 Epstein-Barr virus was shown to be the cause of infectious mononucleosis (IM), or 'glandular fever'. Self-limited conjunctivitis is the most common ocular manifestation of IM, with the reported incidence between less than 1% and 38% (Matoba and McCulley, 1985).

Effective antiviral therapy is available for herpesvirus infections. Aciclovir is effective against HSV and VZV infections, and newer drugs are being evaluated (Wutzler, 1997), while ganciclovir and foscarnet are effective in the treatment of CMV retinitis (Vogel et al, 1997). Prompt laboratory diagnosis allows the selection of an appropriate therapeutic regime. Cell culture, although sensitive, is relatively slow and, at present, one widely used means of rapid diagnosis is the demonstration of viral antigen using highly specific monoclonal antibodies in an immunofluorescence test.

ADENOVIRUSES

In the late 19th century outbreaks of epidemic keratoconjunctivitis (EKC) were described in Austria and Germany. However, 'shipyard eye', as it became known, attracted attention in 1941, when 10,000 shipyard workers in Hawaii were affected. It seemed that the infection was spread by instruments used in the medical facilities for treating workers with eye trauma. Adenoviruses were first cultured in 1953, and in 1955 adenovirus type 8 was identified as the type responsible for 'shipyard eye'. Adenovirus types 19 and 37 have also been shown to cause EKC, which is the most clinically important adenovirus eye infection.

EKC is endemic in large areas of Asia, whilst in Europe and the United States exposure to these types is rare. In developed countries EKC is an iatrogenic disease which can pose an infection-control problem, as demonstrated in two outbreaks in the North of England (Klapper and Cleator, 1995) and a suspected outbreak among operating theatre staff in a Scottish Health trust hospital (*SCIEH Weekly Report*, 1998).

A milder form of adenovirus eye disease is an acute follicular conjunctivitis that can occur separately or as part of a respiratory syndrome, pharyngoconjunctival fever. First described in 1907, it is a self-limiting disease most often seen in children, usually caused by adenovirus type 3, although types 4, 7, and others, have been associated.

So far, antiviral treatment has been generally ineffective. Laboratory diagnosis relies on cell culture and rapid direct immunofluorescence, with molecular-based techniques becoming increasingly used (Klapper and Cleator, 1995).

ENTEROVIRUSES

Some Coxsackie and echoviruses can produce sporadic cases of conjunctivitis: for example, echovirus types 7 and 11, and Coxsackievirus type B2. However, outbreaks of acute haemorrhagic conjunctivitis (AHC) affecting millions of people have been caused by enterovirus type 70 (EV-70) and Coxsackievirus type A24 (C-A24).

Formerly known as Apollo 11 disease, AHC first appeared in 1969 in Ghana. It spread along the west coast of Africa and continued along the north coast, reaching the Middle East and parts of Europe by 1971. AHC occurred mainly in highly populated, humid, coastal cities in the tropics, favouring fomite–finger–eye spread. A new member of the *Picornaviridae*, EV-70, was found to be the cause. Meanwhile an Asian epidemic caused by EV-70 had become established. A painful conjunctivitis with sudden onset, most symptoms resolved within five to 10 days after onset, and the infection was cleared within two to three weeks after onset, with the main ophthalmic sequelae due to bacterial superinfection and the topical administration of steroids. A rare polio-like paralysis occurred in about one case out of 10,000 to 20,000, mostly affecting middle-aged males (Hierholzer and Hatch, 1985).

As the EV-70 epidemic flourished in Asia, an identical disease began in Singapore in the autumn of 1970, which was caused by a variant of C-A24. Unlike EV-70, there were no neurological sequelae associated with AHC due to C-A24 infection. There were also outbreaks involving both EV-70 and C-A24, and, less often, EV-70 and adenovirus (Hierholzer and Hatch, 1985).

Rubella

In 1941 an Australian ophthalmologist, Norman Gregg, related a large outbreak of rubella to the development of congenital cataracts, heart disease and deafness in 78 children of mothers who acquired rubella in early pregnancy. It was soon clear that central nervous system (CNS) involvement occurs, and the so-called 'expanded rubella syndrome" was described, the chief ocular manifestations of which are cataract retinopathy, microphthalmos, glaucoma and corneal cloudiness (Tobin et al, 1977).

Rubella vaccination has seen a decline in the congenital rubella syndrome in the UK. For example, until 1997, 1,103 children had been notified to the National Congenital Rubella Surveillance Programme, which was set up in 1971. In that year 39 new cases were reported; in 1995 there was one case (Miller et al, 1997). Definitive diagnosis of the congenital rubella syndrome is by isolation of the virus, and rubella virus has been grown from an infected lens almost three years after birth (Wolff, 1985). However, the laboratory diagnosis of rubella infection is more often accomplished by serological means, where information on the pre-conception immune status of the mother is important in the interpretation of the results obtained from the mother and/or child.

Poxviruses

With the eradication of smallpox, widespread vaccination with vaccinia virus has stopped. However, the recent use of vaccinia virus in gene transfer experiments means that specialised groups may be exposed to the virus and require vaccination. Accidental auto-inoculation of the eye from the vaccination site may occur, often affecting the eyelid, although there may be keratitis, and conjunctival and corneal involvement.

Molluscum contagiosum is a benign tumour affecting only humans. It is spread by direct and indirect contact, and occurs more often in children than adults, although it is increasingly seen as a sexually transmitted disease among young adults. Eye involvement consists chiefly of molluscum of the eyelids. In HIV-positive patients, molluscum contagiosum is commoner and more severe than in HIV-negative patients, and eyelid involvement is found in up to 5% of HIV-positive individuals (Bardenstein, cited in Cunningham and Margolis, 1998).

Poxvirus particles can be detected by electron microscopy.

Orthomyxoviruses

In the course of studying seals who died of haemorrhagic pneumonia caused by influenza A, some marine biologists contracted a painful, purulent conjunctivitis (Webster et al, 1981). The rare cases of acute conjunctivitis which may be seen during influenza epidemics are probably due to secondary bacterial infection, while anterior uveitis is the most common ocular complication of influenza (Schlaegel and Grayson, 1985).

Paramyxoviruses

Some infections by members of the rubulavirus and the morbillivirus genera of the *Paramyxoviridae* family may have ocular manifestations.

Mumps virus is a member of the rubulavirus genus, and following the onset of parotitis during mumps, the eyes may be one of several organs symptomatically involved (Wolinsky, 1996). Dacryoadenitis, the most common manifestation, is normally bilateral and usually heals completely (Darrell, 1985b). Another rubulavirus, Newcastle disease virus (NDV), was first isolated on a farm near Newcastle-upon-Tyne, and causes a serious and often fatal disease of poultry worldwide, with attendant economic consequences. Laboratory workers handling NDV are at risk of contracting conjunctivitis, as are poultry workers and veterinary surgeons working with infected flocks (Darrell, 1985c).

The eye involvement in classic measles, a morbillivirus infection, is a mild keratoconjunctivitis, which, together with fever, coryza and cough, typically precedes the characteristic maculopapular rash. Occasionally corneal ulceration occurs, and measles retinopathy is a rare complication. In developing countries, the problem of post-measles blindness is caused by measles keratoconjunctivitis being exacerbated by poor nutrition and inappropriate treatment with traditional medical preparations. Subacute sclerosing panencephalitis (SSPE) is a rare degenerative disease of the central nervous system related to infection with measles virus (Morgan and Rapp, 1977). Because of the widespread CNS involvement in SSPE, there is a high incidence of eye involvement in affected patients, which includes papilledema, optic atrophy and disruption of eye movement.

Papovaviruses

The papillomavirinae are a sub-family of the *Papovaviridae*. Commonly known as warts, there are at least 83 different types which can infect the skin, mouth, the aerodigestive tract and the anogenital tract. Human papillomaviruses types 6 and 11 cause most of the rare childhood conjunctival papillomas, and some of the equally rare adult ones (Shah and Howley, 1996).

The polyomavirinae are the second *Papovaviridae* sub-family, and are mainly associated with disease in the immunocompromised. Progressive multifocal leucoencephalopathy (PML) is a rare progressive demyelinating disease of the CNS caused by JC virus, which was first isolated in 1971 from the brain of a PML patient. The AIDS era has seen an increase in the number of reports of PML, the main ocular manifestation of which is visual impairment, often rapidly progressing to blindness.

Retroviruses

This family contains the lentivirus genus, of which HIV is a member. Of the 30 million plus HIV-positive individuals worldwide, between 70% and 80%, mostly adults, will be affected by an HIV-related eye disorder (Cunningham and Margolis, 1998).

Between 50% and 70% of HIV-positive individuals will be affected by retinal microvasculopathy, or HIV retinopathy, characterised by cotton-wool spots, intraretinal haemorrhages and retinal microaneurysms, while between 10% and 20% of patients will experience keratoconjunctivitis sicca, a probable consequence of HIV-mediated inflammation (Cunningham and Margolis, 1998). Less common manifestations include Kaposi's sarcoma of the eyelid or conjunctiva, and ocular toxoplasmosis.

REFERENCES

Arvin, A. (1996) Varicella-zoster virus. In: Fields, B. N., Knipe, D. M., Howley, P. M. et al (eds) *Fields Virology*. Philadelphia: Lippincott-Raven, 3rd edn.

Cunningham, E. T., Margolis, T. P. (1998) Ocular manifestations of HIV infection. *New England Journal of Medicine*; 339: 3, 236–243.

Darougar, S., Treharne, J. D., Monnickendam, M. A. (1985) Herpes simplex virus infections of the eye. In: Waterson, A. P. (ed.) *Recent Advances in Clinical Virology Number 2*. Edinburgh: Churchill Livingstone.

Darrell, R. W. (1985a) Introduction. In: Darrell, R. W. (ed.) *Viral Diseases of the Eye*. Philadelphia: Lea & Febiger.

Darrell, R. W. (1985b) Mumps virus ocular disease. In: Darrell, R. W. (ed.) *Viral Diseases of the Eye*. Philadelphia: Lea & Febiger.

Darrell, R. W. (1985c) Newcastle disease virus ocular infections. In: Darrell, R. W. (ed.) *Viral Diseases of the Eye*. Philadelphia: Lea & Febiger.

Gillies, M., Donovan, B. (1998) Ophthalmology and sexual health medicine. *International Journal of STD and AIDS*; 9: 311–317.

Hierholzer, J. C., Hatch, M. H. (1985) Acute hemorrhagic conjunctivitis. In: Darrell, R. W. (ed.) *Viral Diseases of the Eye*. Philadelphia: Lea & Febiger.

Ives, D. V. (1997) Cytomegalovirus disease in AIDS. *AIDS*; 11: 1791–1797.

Klapper, P. E., Cleator, G. M. (1995) Adenovirus cross-infection: a continuing problem. *Journal of Hospital Infection*; 30: suppl., 262–267.

LaRocco, M. T., Burgert, S. J. (1997) Infection in the bone marrow transplant recipient and role of the microbiology laboratory in clinical transplantation. *Clinical Microbiology Reviews*; 10: 2, 277–297.

McCartney, R. A., Howe, I., Bell, F., Clements, G. B. (1998) The routine use of the Ligase Chain Reaction (LCR) in the laboratory diagnosis of genital *Chlamydia trachomatis* infections: a 12 month study. *SCIEH Weekly Report*; 32: 98/37, 201–202.

Marsh, R. J. (1985) Ophthalmic herpes zoster. In: Darrell, R. W. (ed.) *Viral Diseases of the Eye*. Philadelphia: Lea & Febiger.

Matoba, A. Y., McCulley, J. M. (1985) Epstein-Barr virus and its ocular manifestations. In: Darrell, R. W. (ed.) *Viral Diseases of the Eye*. Philadelphia: Lea & Febiger.

Miller, E., Waight, P., Gay, N. et al (1997) The epidemiology of rubella in England and Wales before and after the 1994 measles and rubella vaccination campaign: fourth joint report from the PHLS and the National Congenital Rubella Surveillance Programme. *CDR Review*; 7: 2, 26–32.

Morgan, E. M., Rapp, F. (1977) Measles virus and its associated diseases. *Bacteriological Reviews*; 41: 3, 636–666.

Schachter, J., Ridgway, G. L., Collier, L. (1998) Chlamydial diseases. In: Hausler, W. J., Sussman, M. (eds) *Topley and Wilson's Microbiology and Microbial Infections*, vol. 3: *Bacterial Infections*. London: Arnold.

Schlaegel, T. F., Grayson, M. L. (1985) Orthomyxoviridae. In: Darrell, R. W. (ed.) *Viral Diseases of the Eye*. Philadelphia: Lea & Febiger.

SCIEH Weekly Report (1998) Outbreak of suspected 'shipyard eye' in Forth Valley; 31: 98/04, 17.

Shah, K. V., Howley, P. M. (1996) Papillomaviruses. In: Fields, B. N., Knipe, D. M., Howley, P. M. et al (eds) *Fields Virology*. Philadelphia: Lippincott-Raven, 3rd edn.

Tobin, J. O'H., Marshall, W. C., Peckham, C. S. (1977) Virus infections. *Clinics in Obstetrics and Gynaecology*; 4: 479–501.

Uchida, Y. (1985) Varicella dendritic keratitis. In: Darrell, R. W. (ed.) *Viral Diseases of the Eye*. Philadelphia: Lea & Febiger.

Vogel, J., Scholz, M., Cinatl, J. (1997) Treatment of cytomegalovirus diseases. *Intervirology*; 40: 357–367.

Webster, R. G., Geraci, J. R., Petursson, G., Skirnisson, K. (1981) Conjunctivitis in human beings caused by influenza A virus of seals. *New England Journal of Medicine*; 304: 911.

Wolff, S. M. (1985) Rubella syndrome. In: Darrell, R. W. (ed.) *Viral Diseases of the Eye*. Philadelphia: Lea & Febiger.

Wolinsky, J. S. (1996) Mumps virus. In: Fields, B. N., Knipe, D. M., Howley, P. M. et al (eds) *Fields Virology*. Philadelphia: Lippincott-Raven, 3rd edn.

Wutzler, P. (1997) Antiviral therapy of herpes simplex and varicella-zoster virus infections. *Intervirology;* 40: 343–356.

10 Pregnancy

Some are born to sweet delight,
Some are born to endless night.

William Blake (1757–1827), 'Auguries of Innocence'.

The immune system exists to maintain the integrity of the body by destroying foreign antigens. These may be from without: for example, viruses, bacteria and parasites; or within: for example, tumour cells and transplantation antigens. Simplified, the two main components of the immune system comprise B lymphocytes, concerned with the antibody response, and T lymphocytes, concerned with cell-mediated immunity (CMI). However, other types of cells are marshalled during the immune response. For example, certain macrophages, together with polymorphonuclear phagocytes, are involved in the direct eating and digestion (phagocytosis) of microbes, while others 'process' antigens in order to present them to immune lymphocytes. In addition, natural killer (NK) cells are lymphocytes which have a role in defence against intracellular pathogens, especially herpesviruses.

During pregnancy, Dad's antigenic contribution to the foetus makes it seem 'foreign' to Mum's immune system, yet the foetus and placenta are not rejected. It seems that there is a non-specific reduction in the maternal immune response that protects the foetus from immunising the mother. This reduction appears to take the form of a natural depression of CMI during pregnancy, one result of which may be an increased susceptibility to infection (Gall, 1977).

Compared to the general public, pregnant women with young families are exposed to many of the common viruses. Although the 'immunosuppressive' effect of pregnancy may increase the risk of maternal infection, various mechanisms protect the foetal immune system from antigenic challenge. There is the mechanical barrier of the mother's skin; contiguous with this are the mucosal surfaces of the maternal respiratory, gastrointestinal and genitourinary tracts, enhanced by the presence of secretory immunoglobulin (Ig) A. Phagocytic cells may also be present on or in the mucosae.

If a virus breaches these defences, it is faced with various non-specific cellular determinants of innate immunity such as tissue macrophages or polymorphonuclear leucocytes. These cells are suspended in a chemical environment, which is generally unfavourable to microbes and exists regardless of the infectious challenge.

If the virus persists, it may evoke a classical immune response in the mother. Additionally, certain T lymphocytes may be stimulated to produce interferons, helping to prevent the virus spreading. However, in a pregnant mother with no prior antigenic experience of the virus, the foetus may be reached before an effective maternal response has been mounted.

The maternal and foetal circulations are in close contact in the placenta, but the barrier is not absolute. If a virus is present in the maternal bloodstream, it may cross the placenta directly, or infect the placenta before reaching the foetus. Most intrauterine infections acquired from the maternal bloodstream are viral rather than bacterial (Larsen and Galask, 1977). Having reached the foetus, the virus will encounter any innate foetal immunity and, perhaps, evoke a foetal immune response. However, the foetus is at risk of infection from other microbial diseases. For example, *Toxoplasma gondii* and *Treponema pallidum* cause congenital infections, haemolytic streptococci group B cause premature delivery and stillbirth, and *Listeria monocytogenes* may cause miscarriage and pre-term delivery (Remington and Klein, 1995).

The effects of transplacentally acquired intrauterine virus infection in live-borne infants include:

- normal infants (However, absence of clinical disease in the newborn does not preclude abnormalities manifesting themselves as the child develops. For example, hearing defects discovered years after birth may be the only outcome of congenital rubella infection.)
- prematurity
- intrauterine growth retardation and low birth weight
- developmental abnormalities

- congenital disease
- persistent postnatal infection

Intrauterine infection with rubella, cytomegalovirus (CMV), varicella zoster virus (VZV), human parvovirus B19, human immunodeficiency virus (HIV) and *Toxoplasma gondii* may follow maternal infection. *Toxoplasma gondii* (a protozoan) is included here because the laboratory diagnosis of toxoplasmosis is often undertaken in diagnostic virology laboratories.

At delivery, herpes simplex virus (HSV), CMV, HIV, VZV, hepatitis B virus (HBV), hepatitis C virus (HCV), enteroviruses, human T-cell lymphotropic viruses (HTLV-1 and 2) and human papillomaviruses (HPV) may be acquired.

Perinatal acquisition of HBV, HCV, HIV and HTLVs can result in persistent infection and chronic disease. HBV, HCV and HIV are blood-borne infections; HTLVs are transmitted in breast milk.

Rubella

'German', as in German measles, or rubella, probably derives from the Old French *germane*, which is derived from *germanus*, meaning 'closely akin to'. So, German measles means 'similar to measles', which, in some respects, it is (Asaad and Ljungars-Esteves, 1985). Rubella was considered an unimportant childhood infection until 1941, when it attracted the attention of an Australian ophthalmic surgeon, Norman Gregg. He noticed that an unusually high number of infants with congenital cataracts and other abnormalities were born in Sydney, and elsewhere in Australia. Gregg also observed that in nearly all cases, their mothers had contracted rubella in the first three months of pregnancy, during a widespread epidemic of the disease.

These observations were confirmed elsewhere, and the isolation of rubella virus in 1962 enabled patterns of excretion and antibody responses to be defined. Rubella is caused by an enveloped, RNA-containing virus which belongs to the *Togaviridae* family. The rubella pandemic which swept the United States and western Europe in 1963–65 unfortunately resulted in large numbers of affected infants, which enabled the natural history of congenital rubella to be defined and stimulated work on a vaccine. By 1965 vaccine trials had begun in the United States, and in 1970 a rubella vaccine was available in the UK.

The earlier non-immune women become infected during pregnancy, the greater the risk of foetal damage. Rubella infection during the first eight weeks of pregnancy may result in spontaneous abortion in up to 20% of cases (Best and O'Shea, 1995). Maternal rubella in the first 12 weeks of pregnancy carries a 90% risk of congenital abnormalities occurring (Table 10.1). Manifestations of congenital rubella include:

- microcephaly and cerebral palsy
- cataract and retinopathy
- hepatosplenomegaly
- deafness
- congenital heart disease
- minor degrees of mental retardation (Tobin et al, 1977)

Virus infection	Maternal infection (weeks gestation)	Rate of transmission to fetus	Risk of congenital abnormalities in those infected
Rubella	1–12	90%	90%
	13–16		~ 17%
Cytomegalovirus	1–40	30–40%	10%
Varicella	1–12		0.4%
	13–20	13–50%[a]	2.0%
Parvovirus B19	1–40	33%	Nil[b]
HIV	Persistent	27%	Nil

[a] from Enders et al, 1994
[b] Approximate 9% risk of spontaneous abortion

Table 10.1 Risk of intrauterine virus infections

Source: Reprinted from *Clinical and Diagnostic Virology*, 5, J. M. Best, Laboratory diagnosis of intrauterine and perinatal virus infections, pp. 121–129. © 1996, with permission from Elsevier Science

Maternal infection between the 13th and 16th weeks of gestation carries a 17% risk of congenital abnormalities occurring in those infected (Best, 1996). Infection after 16 weeks of gestation is not usually associated with defects, although deafness has occurred after infection at 22 weeks' gestation (Tobin et al, 1977).

The first priority of rubella vaccination is to protect the population currently at risk – women of childbearing age. In 1970–71 a rubella vaccination programme began in the UK aimed at schoolgirls aged between 10 and 14 years and at all susceptible women of childbearing age. As a result of vaccination the epidemiology of rubella has changed, vaccination strategies have evolved to meet these changes, and vaccination has been a success, with only about 2% of women of childbearing age being susceptible to rubella infection (Miller et al, 1997) and a dramatic fall in the incidence of congenital rubella (Table 10.2).

Year of	**Congenital rubella**		
birth	**syndrome**	**infection only**	**Unclassified**
Pre-1971	73	4	83
1971	39	5	19
1972	45	6	32
1973	55	12	26
1974	28	6	18
1975	34	11	12
1976	26	5	6
1977	11	2	5
1978	43	10	9
1979	68	10	6
1980	24	7	5
1981	10	5	3
1982	28	9	2
1983	49	23	4
1984	35	17	3
1985	17	7	2
1986	24	6	–
1987	29	8	3
1988	18	3	4
1989	8	5	2
1990	9	3	1
1991	3	–	–
1992	7	–	–
1993	1	2	–
1994	7*	–	–
1995	1	–	–
Total	692	166	245

* includes a set of triplets

Table 10.2 Cases reported to the National Congenital Rubella Programme
Source: Reprinted from E. Miller et al (1997). Reproduced with permission of the PHLS Communicable Disease Surveillance Centre, © PHLS

CYTOMEGALOVIRUS

CMV is endemic worldwide, occurs in all populations yet studied, and is the commonest congenital virus infection. However, it is more prevalent in developing countries and among the lower socioeconomic groups of developed countries.

In common with other herpesviruses, following an initial CMV infection, CMV persists in the host by integrating its deoxyribonucleic acid (DNA) into the host DNA, where it remains latent. This latent state may be interrupted from time to time in both children and adults, resulting in virus shedding. CMV can be found in saliva, urine, cervical and vaginal secretions, semen, breast milk, tears, blood and transplanted organs. Infection is usually minor, and no clinically recognised illness is associated with primary exposure to CMV (Jack, 1974), although occasional cases of glandular fever-like illness may occur in immunologically competent individuals. However, CMV may have a major impact if acquired during pregnancy, or during other periods of immunosuppression.

Congenital infection

CMV may be transmitted from mother to infant congenitally or perinatally. Worldwide, CMV congenital infection accounts for about 1% of all live births: that is, one CMV-*infected* infant for every 100 live births. About 10% of infected infants show symptoms of CMV disease (Table 10.3); that is, there is one CMV-*affected* infant for every 1,000 live births (Remington and Klein, 1995). CMV infection can be transmitted to the foetus following a primary infection or the reactivation of a latent infection. The transmission rate of CMV from mother to foetus following a primary infection is about 40% (Fig 10.1). In contrast to rubella (Table 10.1), the transmission rate of congenital CMV is independent of the timing of infection during pregnancy.

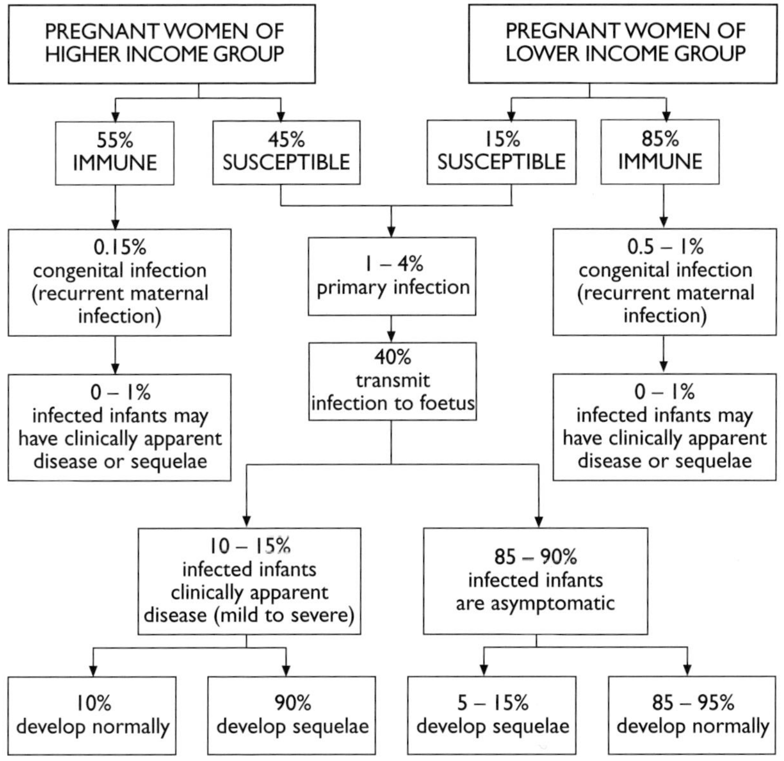

Fig 10.1 Characteristics of cytomegalovirus infection in pregnancy
Source: Reprinted from S. Stagno and R. J. Whitley (1985),

Perinatal infection

This is chiefly the result of mother to child transmission. The two main sources are:

- infected breast milk, which accounts for about 60% of cases of perinatal infection
- the infected genital tract during delivery, which is associated with transmission in between 25% and 50% of cases (WHO Meeting, 1985)

Perinatal infection occurs 10 to 20 times more often than congenital infection, but with minimal clinical symptoms in otherwise healthy infants (Table 10.3).

	Congenital	**Perinatal**
CNS lesions	Deafness Seizures Hydrocephaly Microcephaly Microgyria Periventricular calcification Spastic paralysis Developmental disorders	CNS involvement rare
Other symptoms	Hepatitis Hepatosplenomegaly Hyperbilirubinaemia Thrombocytopenia often with purpura Haemolytic anaemia Chorioretinitis Bronchitis Bronchial pneumonia	Hepatitis Hepatosplenomegaly Thrombocytopenia often with purpura Haemolytic anaemia Pneumonia (sometimes atypical, usually accompanied by Pneumocystis carinii infection
	EBV*-mononucleosis-like syndrome (without heterophilic antibodies)	EBV*-mononucleosis-like syndrome (without heterophilic antibodies)

*Epstein-Barr virus

Table 10.3 Clinical forms of cytomegalovirus infection following congenital and perinatal infection

Source: Adapted with the permission of Dade Behring Ltd, Walton, Milton Keynes MK7 7AJ

VARICELLA

Between approximately 85% and 90% of pregnant women are immune to chickenpox (Carrington et al, 1998). It is estimated that there are 2,000 cases of chickenpox a year in pregnancy in England and Wales (Nathwani et al, 1998). Because adults from the tropics and sub-tropics are more likely to be susceptible to varicella, it is presumed that immigrants, including pregnant women, from these areas who are living in the UK are also more likely to be susceptible to varicella.

Maternal varicella can infect the infant by three routes:

- across the placenta, from the maternal bloodstream
- during birth, from infected lesions in the birth canal or external genitalia
- respiratory transmission and/or direct contact with vesicular lesions after birth

The term foetal varicella syndrome (FVS) is associated with maternal varicella zoster virus (VZV) infection during the first 20 weeks of pregnancy, whereas the term congenital varicella describes intrauterine foetal infection resulting in varicella in the newborn. An infant with chickenpox at 10 days old or less indicates an intrauterine VZV infection, as the incubation period is usually about 14 days.

Congenital abnormalities as a result of FVS include low birth weight, eye defects, neurological abnormalities, and bone and muscle hypoplasia. FVS is very rare (Table 10.1; Enders et al, 1994). In contrast, if a mother develops chickenpox between up to 4 days before delivery and 2 days after delivery, the infant has a 20% risk of congenital chickenpox and a 20–30% risk of death (Nathwani et al, 1998). If an infant acquires chickenpox between 10 and 28 days after birth, it is usually mild.

Aciclovir is currently the only available and approved treatment for varicella in the UK. The role of VZ immunoglobulin and antiviral intervention in prophylaxis and treatment has been recently reviewed for the UK Advisory Group on Chickenpox on behalf of the British Society for the Study of Infection (Ogilvie, 1998).

Parvovirus B19

A member of the family *Parvoviridae*, the DNA virus human parvovirus B19 causes erythema infectiosum (see Chapter 7) and is associated with aplastic crises in patients with diminished red blood cell survival. In 1984 B19 was first recognised as a cause of hydrops foetalis and of intrauterine foetal death.

There is an estimated foetal infection rate of 33%, and an approximate 9% risk of spontaneous abortion occurring (Public Health Laboratory Service Working Party on Fifth Disease, 1990), but no association was found of B19 infection with congenital abnormalities.

HIV

There is an estimated 15% to 20% mother-to-infant transmission rate of HIV infection, and by the end of January 1997, there were 226 cases of such vertically transmitted infection in the UK (Molesworth and Tookey, 1997). Breast-feeding increases the risk of postnatal HIV infection. Most cases of paediatric HIV infection in the UK have been identified in the London area, where most maternal infections are among black Africans who probably acquired HIV abroad through heterosexual exposure. In contrast, in Scotland almost all reported cases of paediatric HIV have been associated with maternal or paternal injecting drug use (Molesworth and Tookey, 1997).

The immunosuppressive effect of pregnancy does not appear to accelerate HIV progression (The European Collaborative Study, 1997). At birth, infants of HIV-infected mothers may not be infected, but will have antibodies to HIV because of transfer of maternal antibodies; their HIV antibody status can only be determined with certainty after 18 months, when maternal antibody should have cleared. If HIV antibody is still present after 18 months, or if there is an AIDS-defining illness or the presence of HIV can be demonstrated, the child is confirmed as HIV-infected.

Herpes simplex virus

Neonatal HSV infection can be acquired in three ways:

- prenatally
- during vaginal delivery
- postnatally

Prenatal infection is uncommon, and symptoms may include hydrocephaly, skin scarring, vesicles and/or chorioretinitis.

Contact with infected maternal genital secretions accounts for between approximately 70% and 80% of cases of neonatal HSV infection (Whitley, 1991). Let us look at maternal HSV infection. In 1996 9,349 women were diagnosed with primary or recurrent genital HSV at genitourinary medicine clinics in England, a 4% rise from 1995, outnumbering men by 2:1, with the highest rates of primary infection occurring in those aged between 20 and 24 years (Simms et al, 1998). At least 85% of all genital HSV infections are caused by HSV type 2 (Whitley, 1991). It is paradoxical that in the UK genital HSV infection in pregnant women is not uncommon, yet neonatal HSV infection is rare. This situation is found in other countries (Remington and Klein, 1995), and it is speculated that an as yet poorly understood mechanism (or mechanisms) protects the foetus (Whitley, 1991).

Almost 30% of neonatal HSV infections are caused by HSV type 1, and while some of these may be acquired during delivery, nosocomial transmission, breast lesions and recurrent cold sores may also have a role (Whitley, 1991).

Neonatal HSV infection is manifested in three main ways:

- skin, eye or mouth involvement
- central nervous system involvement
- disseminated disease

Untreated superficial involvement may lead to disseminated disease in 70% of affected neonates. Intravenous aciclovir is the treatment of choice for suspected or proven neonatal herpes (Krafchik, 1996).

ENTEROVIRUSES

Neonatal enterovirus infections can range from asymptomatic shedding to severe life-threatening disease. Of the enteroviruses, Coxsackie B viruses are most often associated with severe neonatal illness, with myocarditis and/or meningoencephalitis commonly found (Remington and Klein, 1995).

A study in Rochester, New York, of 666 neonates from birth to one month of age, found that enterovirus infection was acquired at a rate of 12.8%, and that most infants were asymptomatic. The risk of enterovirus infection was associated with low socioeconomic status and lack of breast-feeding (Jenista et al, 1984).

LABORATORY DIAGNOSIS AND TORCH

The choice of specimen which is sent to the virus laboratory is determined by each virus. For example, congenital rubella is best diagnosed by the detection of specific IgM in the infant's serum, whereas virus detection in urine is the test of choice for congenital CMV; a clinical or serological diagnosis of congenital VZV is often appropriate, whereas virus detection in vesicular material, nose, throat, eye or mouth swabs, or cerebrospinal fluid (CSF) is favoured for the diagnosis of neonatal HSV infection; enterovirus infections are best diagnosed by the detection of viral ribonucleic acid (RNA); foetal B19 infection is best diagnosed by detection of viral DNA in foetal blood, and serological techniques can diagnose maternal infection with HBV, HCV, HIV and HTLVs.

The use of the acronym and test range encompassed by 'TORCH' should be discouraged. TORCH, devised in 1971, is an acronym for Toxoplasmosis, Other, Rubella, Cytomegalovirus, Herpes. Typically, a serum was submitted for TORCH testing when intrauterine deaths, and congenital, perinatal and neonatal infections were under investigation. TORCH not only excludes many other possible infections, but a serum may be a wholly inappropriate specimen for the investigation of a particular infection. In one study of 603 patients, who underwent TORCH tests during a 4-year period, infection with a TORCH agent was not confirmed serologically in a single patient (Leland et al, 1983).

References

Asaad, F., Ljungars-Esteves, K. (1985) Rubella – world impact. *Reviews of Infectious Diseases*; 7: suppl. 1, S29–S36.

Best, J. M. (1996) Laboratory diagnosis of intrauterine and perinatal virus infections. *Clinical and Diagnostic Virology*; 5: 121–129.

Best, J. M., O'Shea, S. (1995) Rubella virus. In: Lennette, E. H., Lennette, D. A., Lennette, E. T. (eds) *Diagnostic Procedures for Viral, Rickettsial, and Chlamydial Infections*. Washington: American Public Health Association, 7th edn.

Carrington, D., Howard, J., Higson, N. (1998) Summary of questions and answers on chickenpox for primary healthcare personnel. *Journal of Infection*; 36: suppl.1, 79–83.

Enders, G., Miller, E., Cradock-Watson, J. E. et al (1994) Consequences of varicella and herpes zoster in pregnancy: prospective study of 1739 cases. *Lancet*; 343: 1547–1550.

The European Collaborative Study and the Swiss HIV Pregnancy Cohort (1997) Immunological markers in HIV-infected pregnant women. *AIDS*; 11: 1859–1865.

Gall, S. A. (1977) Maternal immune system during human gestation. *Seminars in Perinatology*; 1: 2, 119–133.

Jack, I. (1974) Persistent infections with herpesviruses. *Progress in Medical Virology*; 18, 160–177.

Jenista, J. A., Powell, K. R., Menegus, M. A. (1984) Epidemiology of neonatal enterovirus infection. *Journal of Pediatrics*; 104, 685–690.

Krafchik, B. R. (1996) Advances in viral infections. *Advances in Dermatology*; 11, 155–176.

Larsen, B., Galask, R. P. (1977) Protection of the fetus against infection. *Seminars in Perinatology*; 1: 2, 183–193.

Leland, D., French, M. L. V., Kleiman, M. B., Schreiner, R. L. (1983) The use of TORCH titers. *Pediatrics*; 72: 1, 41–43.

Miller, E., Waight, P., Gay, N. et al (1997) The epidemiology of rubella in England and Wales before and after the 1994 measles and rubella vaccination campaign: fourth joint report from the PHLS and the National Congenital Rubella Surveillance Programme. *CDR Review*; 7: 2, R26–R32.

Molesworth, A., Tookey, P. (1997) Paediatric AIDS and HIV infection. *CDR Review*; 7: 9, R132–R134.

Nathwani, D., Maclean, A., Conway, S., Carrington, D. (1998) Varicella infections in pregnancy and the newborn. *Journal of Infection*; 36: suppl. 1, 59–71.

Ogilvie, M. M. (1998) Antiviral prophylaxis and treatment in chickenpox. *Journal of Infection*; 36: suppl. 1, 31–38.

Public Health Laboratory Service Working Party on Fifth Disease (1990) Prospective study of human parvovirus (B19) infection in pregnancy. *British Medical Journal*; 300: 1166–1170.

Remington, J. S., Klein, J. O. (eds) (1995) *Infectious Diseases of the Fetus and Newborn Infant*. Philadelphia: W. B. Saunders Company, 4th edn.

Simms, I., Hughes, G., Swan, A. V. et al (1998) New cases seen at genitourinary medicine clinics: England 1996. *CDR Supplement*; 8: suppl. 1, S2–S11.

Stagno, S., Whitley, R. J. (1985) Herpesvirus infections of pregnancy. *New England Journal of Medicine;* 313: 1270–1274.

Tobin, J. O'H., Marshall, W. C., Peckham, C. S. (1977) Virus infections. *Clinics in Obstetrics and Gynaecology*; 4: 479–501.

Whitley, R. J. (1991) Perinatal herpes simplex virus infections. *Reviews in Medical Virology*; 1: 101–110.

WHO Meeting (1985) Prevention and control of herpesvirus diseases. Part 2: Epidemiology and immunology. *Bulletin of the World Health Organisation;* 63: 3, 427–444.

11 Hepatitis

> *Those who have ever suffered from a profound derangement of the liver may happen to know that of human despondencies through all their infinite gamut none is more deadly.*
>
> Thomas de Quincey (1785–1859), *Confessions of an English Opium-Eater.*

In 1942 some volunteers were fed the contents of a patient's duodenum. The patient had 'acute catarrhal jaundice', and some time later so did the volunteers, thus demonstrating the infectious nature of the disease. Now called infectious hepatitis, and caused by hepatitis A virus (HAV), the disease has been known for hundreds of years. Also in 1942 30,000 US troops contracted hepatitis, of whom 84 died (Radetsky, 1991). They had all received yellow fever vaccine prepared for soldiers serving in the South Pacific. Unfortunately, human serum had been used as a stabiliser during the vaccine preparation, and it was contaminated with what came to be known as hepatitis B virus (HBV). By 1947, volunteer studies had led to the recognition that there were two manifestations of hepatitis; one a disease associated with unhygienic living conditions, and the other blood-borne. Because no other infectious agent had been found, it was assumed to be viral, but the search for a cause of the disease (or diseases) was hampered by the lack of suitable experimental animals. They were to come from an unexpected, and controversial, source.

In 1956 Saul Krugman, a New York professor of paediatrics, was asked to help solve a worsening problem at the Willowbrook State School, Staten Island. This was an overcrowded home to 4,000 mentally retarded children, among whom hepatitis and other infectious diseases were rife. By the mid-1960s, after experiments which involved both feeding and injecting infected blood into these children, Krugman had discovered that there were indeed two kinds of hepatitis; one spread by the faecal–oral route, and the other by blood and intimate contact which allowed the exchange of body fluids. He designated them MS-1 and MS-2, and they were later named hepatitis A and hepatitis B. The ethics of Krugman's experiments were debated, and even censured by the New York Senate, but there is no doubt that this work represented a watershed in research into viral hepatitis.

At present, the alphabet of viral hepatitis consists of HAV, HBV, hepatitis C (HCV), hepatitis D (HDV), hepatitis E (HEV) and hepatitis G (HGV). HAV and HEV are transmitted enterically, and HBV, HCV, HDV and HGV are transmitted parenterically. The diseases cannot be distinguished clinically and laboratory diagnosis is essential. All six forms can cause acute hepatitis, with some leading to a chronic carrier state.

Hepatitis A

In 1973 prison volunteers were infected with Krugman's MS-1 strain of HAV, and for the first time, the virus was seen by electron microscopy in their stools. Previously described as enterovirus type 72 because of shared characteristics with the enteroviruses, HAV is a non-enveloped virus belonging to the Hepatovirus genus of the *Picornaviridae* family. Like the enteroviruses, HAV is of similar size (27nm–28nm), survives acid conditions and resists the action of ether. Those who enjoy downing a few oysters before windsurfing some of our sewage-laden coastal waters might note that HAV can survive for five days in live oysters, not to mention a 4% survival rate in sea water, while on dry land HAV can survive in dried faeces for a month (Sjogren, 1997).

Transmission is by the faecal–oral route, person-to-person contact, or the ingestion of faecally contaminated food or water, and in the UK hepatitis A is seen as an indicator of urban deprivation. HAV can be transmitted sexually, especially among male homosexuals, but parenteral transmission has only been rarely associated with blood transfusion or the use of blood products. There is an incubation period of 15 to 40 days, with an average of 25 days, and most HAV infections are self-limiting, resolving in one or two months. Asymptomatic infection generally occurs in children under three years of age, but is generally symptomatic and icteric in adults. The risk of HAV transmission is greatest from a fortnight before to a week after the onset of jaundice (Brooks et al, 1991). Hepatitis A has a low mortality of around 0.2%, but may be fatal. For example, of 300,000 individuals in China who had consumed HAV-infected hairy clams, 47 died (*Lancet*, 1990). A vaccine against HAV has been available in Europe since 1992, and high-risk groups to be considered for immunisation include international travellers, active male homosexuals, drug misusers and workers in institutions for people with mental handicap.

In the laboratory acute HAV infection is typically diagnosed by the demonstration of HAV-specific IgM antibody in the patient's serum, using a commercially available enzyme immunoassay (EIA), and is the most reliable marker for determining acute HAV infection. The detection of total antibody to HAV is used to determine previous exposure to the virus.

Hepatitis B

In 1963 Baruch Blumberg, a geneticist at Columbia medical school in New York, found that the blood of some haemophilia patients contained antibodies which reacted with an antigen in the serum of an Australian aborigine. He called it the Australia antigen, known today as hepatitis B surface antigen (HBsAg), and showed that it is a marker for the presence of HBV. For this, Blumberg was awarded a Nobel prize in 1976.

HBV is a deoxyribonucleic acid (DNA) virus of the *Hepadnaviridae* family. The virus is 42nm in size, and consists of a circle of DNA inside a 27nm inner core (HBcAg) surrounded by an envelope of HBsAg. The HBV DNA is unique in that it is partly single-stranded and partly double-stranded. During HBV infection, both complete and incomplete virus particles are produced. Incomplete particles have no core nor DNA, but consist entirely of HBsAg. For every complete virus, there may be up to one million incomplete particles. A third component of HBV is the hepatitis B e antigen (HBeAg), which is associated with the HBcAg part of the virus. As HBeAg denotes the presence of complete virus, it is a reliable marker of infectivity.

HBV is found worldwide, where there are 400 million carriers. The prevalence of HBsAg varies from less than 0.5% in developed countries, such as the UK, Canada and USA, to between 5% and 20% in parts of China, Africa and South America (Hollinger, 1996).

Susceptible adults can acquire a primary HBV infection from parenteral exposure to infected blood, or blood products, or from sexual contact with an infected host; the incubation period is between 30 and 150 days. HBV is often spread by blood transfusion, the injection of blood products, accidental needlestick injuries, tattooing and body-piercing, and the sharing of needles by drug misusers; while perinatal and transplacental transmission may contribute to the pool of HBV carriers worldwide. However, sexual transmission is common, especially among male homosexuals and among prostitutes.

Primary infection can be asymptomatic or may result in acute hepatitis, which has a mortality rate of between 0.2% and 2%. The primary infection is often cleared, but a persistent infection will arise in about 5% of adults. Although many such persistently infected individuals are asymptomatic, they constitute the main reservoir from which susceptible hosts become infected. Persistently infected patients are at an increased risk of developing hepatocellular carcinoma, and there is substantial evidence for a causal link between HBV infection and this cancer.

There is an effective vaccine against HBV, which is currently available in the UK for certain at-risk groups and which reduces the risk of healthcare workers acquiring HBV from patients. Though infrequent, nosocomial transmission from infected healthcare workers to patients can occur. In 1981 official guidelines (Department of Health, 1981) stated that no restrictions should be placed on the clinical duties undertaken by HBV carriers, the exception being that HBV carriers should not work in renal dialysis units. Meanwhile, outbreaks of HBV infection caused by healthcare workers continued, and in the UK debate grew as to whether surgeons who are HbeAg-positive should be allowed to perform exposure-prone procedures (Cockroft and Walker, 1991), eventually leading to restrictions on the procedures which could be performed by HbeAg-positive workers (UK Health Departments, 1993). However, since a report of the death of a woman after HBV transmission from an HbeAg-negative surgeon (Sundkvist et al, 1998), current guidelines may need to be reconsidered.

The most widely used test for the laboratory diagnosis of HBV infection is the detection of HBsAg, for which many sensitive commercial screening EIAs are available. During acute HBV infection, high concentrations of HBsAg can be found in the serum, but the concentration of HBsAg may vary in the sera of chronic carriers. Tests for the presence of other hepatitis B markers are available to monitor the course of clinical disease in a patient, including the detection of antibody to HBsAg (anti-HBs), which is also widely used as part of the follow-up to HBV vaccination (Cameron, 1997).

Hepatitis C

By 1975 laboratory tests to identify HAV and HBV infection became available, but by the 1980s it was clear that most cases of post-transfusion hepatitis were caused by neither HAV nor HBV. Such hepatitis was originally referred to as non-A, non-B hepatitis, but most is now known to be caused by a further virus, HCV.

Using chimpanzees as an animal model, it was found in 1983 that the presumptive virus was sensitive to chloroform treatment, and thus contained a lipid envelope. However, further progress was limited. It seemed that as the conventional methods of trying to grow the virus, or identify it by immunological means, were unsuccessful, a novel approach might help. It was the application of relatively recently discovered molecular cloning techniques to the plasma of chimpanzees infected with non-A, non-B hepatitis which led to the discovery of the HCV genome in 1989. It seems remarkable that the nucleic acid of HCV was identified before the other components of the virus. An RNA virus, it is now classified as a Hepacivirus in the *Flaviviridae* family

HCV infection is worldwide, with an estimated 350 million infected individuals (Brechot and Pol, 1997). In South America, parts of Africa and the Middle East, up to 10% of the population might be chronically infected, whereas in the UK, prevalence is less than 2% (Ramsay et al, 1998). HCV is most commonly transmitted by blood transfusion, exposure to blood or blood products, needlestick injuries and parenteral drug abuse. Mother-to-child transmission probably occurs, with an incidence of between 5% and 10% (Van der Poel, 1994), while firm evidence of sexual transmission is awaited. In the UK blood donations have been screened for antibody to HCV since 1991, and it is estimated that in England the risk of an HCV-infected donation entering the blood supply is one in more than 200,000 (Ramsay et al, 1998).

The incubation period of hepatitis C ranges from 15 to 120 days, with a mean of 50 days. The main feature of HCV infection is its chronicity (60% to 80%) and the risk of chronic active hepatitis, cirrhosis and hepatocellular carcinoma. The mortality of hepatitis C ranges from 0.2% to 2%.

Laboratory diagnosis of HCV infection is based on the detection of antibody to HCV using an EIA. In addition, the polymerase chain reaction (PCR) can be used to detect the presence of HCV RNA to help determine whether the infection is active. Treatment with interferon and ribavirin has given encouraging results, and we can expect that the measurement of the amount of circulating RNA, or viral load, will assume increasing importance as more refined and effective treatments become available.

Hepatitis D

In 1977 Mario Rizetto, an Italian gastroenterologist, discovered hepatitis delta virus (HDV) while studying patients with chronic HBV infection. Not all HBsAg-positive patients have HDV infection, but all patients with HDV infection are HBsAg positive, and tend to have the most severe forms of acute and chronic hepatitis. HDV is a unique RNA virus which only infects cells already infected with HBV, a DNA virus. Once inside the cell, HDV RNA directs the production of delta protein, but instead of making its own virus coat, HDV simply pushes into the hepatitis B production line and steals the HBV coat for itself. Although it is now designated as a hepatitis virus, HDV may have evolved from viroids, which consist of a single rod-like molecule of RNA and are associated with many plant diseases. With a mean incubation period of 35 days, the mortality rate of hepatitis D is between 2% and 20%. Transmission of HDV is by exposure to blood, or blood products or close personal contact, and HDV is particularly prevalent in the Middle East, the Amazon and Mediterranean basins, and Central Asia. Vaccination against HBV will also control HDV infections. In the UK the laboratory diagnosis of HDV infection is presently confined to specialised laboratories and is not widely available.

Hepatitis E

In New Delhi in 1955, almost 30,000 cases of icteric hepatitis occurred after faecal contamination of the drinking-water system. Originally thought to be caused by HAV, retrospective serological tests showed that neither HAV nor HBV could be implicated. Hepatitis E has also been called *enterically transmitted non-A, non-B hepatitis*, and, like hepatitis A, is a self-limiting disease with no chronicity. HEV infection is typically associated with large waterborne epidemics in developing countries. The mortality rate is between 0.2% and 1%. However, one major difference with HAV is that in pregnant women infected with HEV, there is a strikingly high mortality rate of up to 20% (Purcell, 1996).

HEV is an RNA virus, 32nm in size, belonging to the family *Caliciviridae*. It is usually spread by faecally contaminated water, but, unlike HAV, is rarely transmitted beyond the index case. It is thought that the very low secondary attack rate among household contacts may be due to the relative instability of HEV (Krawczynski, 1993). The incubation period of hepatitis E is 20 to 55 days, with an average of 40 days. In the UK HEV infection is usually seen only in patients who have returned from endemic areas. For example, during the first half of 1998, there were seven laboratory reports of hepatitis E in England and Wales, compared with 379 reports of hepatitis A and 1,138 reports of hepatitis C (*CDR Weekly*, 1998). Serological diagnosis using commercial EIAs for the detection of IgG and/or IgM is available in some reference laboratories, where they can help in the differential diagnosis of acute hepatitis in patients who have returned from endemic areas.

Hepatitis G

With hepatitis viruses A, B, C, D and E established, the search for hepatitis F continued apace. Some researchers thought they had found it, and then it seemed they hadn't. Whatever, there was some confusion, and when the next candidate hepatitis virus arose, it was decided, for clarity, not to call it hepatitis F. Hepatitis G was chosen instead. However, some think that the designation 'hepatitis' G might be imprecise, as there is only slowly mounting evidence that hepatitis G virus (HGV) actually causes anything. However, the story behind the virus is interesting (Hadziyannis, 1997).

In the 1960s, a 34-year-old surgeon from Chicago developed acute hepatitis of unknown origin. His initials were GB. Some of GB's serum was injected into monkeys, who later showed evidence of hepatitis. Surprisingly, the GB agent (or agents) received no more attention until 1995, when researchers at Abbott Laboratories began working with stored monkey serum samples from the original GB experiments and isolated a virus they termed GBV-C. However, they were unable to detect GBV-C in GB's original stored serum. They had identified a virus originating from the GB experiments, which was nevertheless unrelated to the hepatitis which GB had in the first place.

Meanwhile, independently, a group working for Genelabs Technologies identified a virus in the plasma of a patient with chronic hepatitis and called it HGV. It is now recognised that GBV-C and HGV are independent isolates of the same virus. HGV is an RNA virus in the same Hepacivirus group as HCV in the *Flaviviridae* family, and is distantly related to HCV.

HGV seems to be spread mainly by parenteral transmission of contaminated blood and blood products, and occurs among multiply transfused patients, haemophiliacs, and intravenous drug abusers who share needles and syringes. Disease seems to be asymptomatic, transient and self-limiting, giving rise to the suggestion that HGV is an 'accidental tourist' that just happens to be there, an orphan in search of a parent disease (Hadziyannis, 1997). However, there is evidence that HGV is involved in some cases of acute and chronic hepatitis, and that it replicates in the human liver, suggesting that the designation 'hepatitis' G may be appropriate after all (Mushahwar and Zuckerman, 1998).

It is unlikely that the hepatitis alphabet is complete, as the recent Japanese discovery of a transfusion-transmissible DNA virus, possibly a parvovirus, illustrates. However, while its global distribution has been confirmed (Simmonds et al, 1998), caution has been urged as to whether we should actually consider it as a pathogen, at this stage (Cossart, 1998).

References

Brechot, C., Pol, S. (1997) Hepatitis C virus biology and genetic variability: implications for the management of infected patients. *Progress in Liver Diseases*; 15: 183–217.

Brooks, G. F., Butel, J. S., Ornston, L. N. (1991) Hepatitis viruses. In: *Jawetz, Melnick & Adelberg's Medical Microbiology*. East Norwalk, CT: Appleton & Lange.

Cameron, S. O. (1997) Diagnostic perspective of viral hepatitis. *Reviews in Medical Microbiology*; 8: 4, 197–207.

CDR Weekly (1998) Viral hepatitis, England and Wales: laboratory reports, weeks 16–19/98; 8: 20, 177.

Cockroft, A., Walker, P. (1991) Surgeons who test positive for the e antigen of hepatitis B should be transferred to low-risk duties. *Reviews in Medical Virology*; 1: 195–200.

Cossart, Y. (1998) TTV a common virus, but pathogenic? *Lancet*; 352: 164.

Department of Health (1981) Chief Medical Officer's Letter. London: DoH 1981(CMO (81) 11).

Hadziyannis, S. J. (1997) The 'hepatitis' G virus: biology, epidemiology, and search for disease. *Progress in Liver Diseases*; 15: 219–245.

Hollinger, F. B. (1996) Hepatitis B virus. In: Fields, B. N., Knipe, D. M., Howley, P. M. et al (eds) *Fields Virology*, Philadelphia: Lippincott-Raven, 3rd edn.

Krawczynski, K. (1993) Hepatitis E. *Hepatology*; 17: 932–941.

Lancet (1990) The A to F of viral hepatitis (editorial); 336: 8724, 1158–1160.

Mushahwar, I. K., Zuckerman, J. N. (1998) Clinical implications of GB virus C. *Journal of Medical Virology*; 56: 1–3.

Purcell, R. H. (1996) Hepatitis E virus. In: Fields, B. N., Knipe, D. M., Howley, P. M. et al (eds) *Fields Virology*. Philadelphia: Lippincott-Raven, 3rd edn.

Radetsky, P. (1991) *The Invisible Invaders: The Story of the Emerging Age of Viruses*. Boston: Little, Brown & Co.

Ramsay, M. E., Balogun, M. A., Collins, M., Balraj, V. (1998) Laboratory surveillance of hepatitis C virus infection in England and Wales: 1992 to 1996. *Communicable Disease and Public Health*; 1: 2, 89–94.

Simmonds, P., Davidson, F., Lycett, C. et al (1998) Detection of a novel DNA virus (TTV) in blood donors and blood products. *Lancet*; 352: 191–194.

Sjogren, M. H. (1997) Hepatitis A virus. *Progress in Liver Diseases*; 15: 171–181.

Sundkvist, T., Hamilton, G. R., Rimmer, D. et al (1998) Fatal outcome of transmission of hepatitis B from an e antigen negative surgeon. *Communicable Disease and Public Health*; 1: 1, 48–50.

UK Health Departments (1993) Protecting health care workers and patients from hepatitis B: recommendations of the Advisory Group on Hepatitis. London: HMSO.

Van der Poel, C. L. (1994) Hepatitis C virus: epidemiology, transmission and prevention. In: Reesink, H. W. (ed) *Hepatitis C Virus* (Current Studies in Hematology and Blood Transfusion, no. 61). Basle: Karger.

12 Transplantation

He who helps in the saving of others,
Saves himself as well.

Hartmann von Aue (*c.* 1170–1215), 'Poor Henry'.

Kidney, heart, lung, liver, cornea, bone marrow; their transplantation has become a standard therapeutic option for several end-stage organ dysfunctions and for certain malignancies. Pancreas and small-bowel transplantations are increasing, and the world's first human laryngeal transplant was carried out in 1998 (Birchall, 1998). Improvements in medical management and surgical technique, combined with progress in immunosuppressive therapy, have contributed to the success of transplantation medicine, which continues to expand – as do waiting lists (Table 12.1), and in the UK research on xenotransplantation looks set to continue under the guidance of the UK Xenotransplantation Interim Regulatory Authority, which considers problems such as the issue of retroviruses in potential porcine organ donors.

Year	Liver transplants	Liver waiting list
1987	177	–
1988	244	–
1989	298	–
1990	359	57
1991	421	83
1992	508	83
1993	551	119
1994	644	115
1995	657	153
1996	652	195
1997	696	196

Table 12.1 Liver transplants in the UK and the Republic of Ireland 1987–97
Source: Statistics prepared by the UK Transplant Support Service Authority from the National Transplant Database maintained on behalf of the UK transplant community

Infection is the main cause of death in transplant patients. As more transplants are performed with improved survival rates, infection in recipients represents an increasing challenge for the future. This problem is particularly acute for diagnostic laboratory services, on which demands for accurate, timely results will be made against a background of economic constraints.

Clearly, consultation between the nurse, clinician and relevant laboratories is important in evaluating the risks posed to the transplant patient by bacteria, fungi, parasites and viruses. Changes to laboratory testing protocols can mean different, and often more rigorous, requirements in the way that specimens are collected and/or stored if tests are to have meaningful results. Such requirements place additional demands on nursing staff to comply with protocols, which seem to the outsider unduly stringent. For example, effective viral load testing for cytomegalovirus (CMV) depends on appropriately collected and stored specimens being taken on the ward, and received by the laboratory within a certain time limit so as to maintain the viability of viral nucleic acids. It is likely that cooperation between ward and laboratory will increase (near-patient testing is already commonplace), and a broadening of nurses' training base to include more microbiology may be useful.

Vaccinations are an important part of the prospective recipient's pre-transplant work-up. Hepatitis B, influenza and inactivated polio vaccines should be given to unvaccinated candidates. However, the role of live vaccines, such as measles and varicella, is more problematic (Patel and Paya, 1997).

In the pre-transplant serological screening of recipient and donor, it is important to detect evidence of past as well as current infection (Table 12.2). Active infection in a prospective recipient could delay a transplant: similarly, evidence of a latent or active infection in a prospective donor may prevent the organ from being used. It is especially important to have evidence of latent or active infection with members of the herpesvirus family. For example, if the prospective recipient is seronegative for CMV, CMV-negative blood products are usually indicated; a varicella zoster virus (VZV) negative individual might need VZV vaccine to obviate the risk of a severe primary varicella infection. When a donor is seropositive for CMV and/or Epstein-Barr virus (EBV), this should alert clinicians to the risk of these viruses reactivating in the recipient at some time after transplant.

History

Immunosuppressive therapy: type and duration (current or past)
Antibiotic allergies: probable or documented
Past medical history: infectious diseases
- Oral: dental caries, sinusitis, pharyngitis, HSV infection
- Respiratory: pneumonia, tuberculosis
- Cardiovascular: valvular heart disease, heart murmur (need for endocarditis prophylaxis)
- Gastrointestinal: diverticulitis, diarrheal disease, hepatitis A, B, or C, intestinal parasitic infection
- Genitourinary: urinary tract infections, prostatitis, vaginitis, genital herpes, genital warts, syphilis, gonorrhea, pelvic inflammatory disease, chlamydial infection
- Cutaneous: skin and nail infections, varicella, and zoster
- Osteoarticular: osteomyelitis, prosthetic joint(s)
- Childhood illnesses: chicken pox, measles, rubella
- Other: mononucleosis, other infectious diseases not included above

Exposure history
- Travel history: prior residence in or travel to areas associated with the geographically restricted endemic mycoses and/or parasitic disease, especially *S. stercoralis,* malaria, etc.
- Tuberculosis: exposure, prior tuberculous skin testing, chest x-ray abnormality
- Risk factors for blood-borne pathogen infection (including HIV)
- Animal and pet exposure (including vaccination status of pets); *Brucella* exposure
- Occupational exposure: farming, animal husbandry, gardening
- Drinking-water source
- Exposure to young children
- Dietary habits: consumption of raw meat, unpasteurized milk products, and seafood

Physical examination

Infectious-diseases testing

Tuberculin skin test and limited energy panel
Chest and sinus x-rays
Urine analysis and culture for bacteria
Stool culture and examination for ova and parasites
Serologic tests: CMV, VZV, EBV, HSV, *T. gondii,* syphilis, HBV, HCV, HIV (geographically restricted endemic mycoses if history of exposure present)

Vaccinations
Tetanus-diphtheria (update)
Influenza
Pneumococcus
Hepatitis B
H. influenzae type b (pediatric patients)
Inactivated polio vaccine

Table 12.2 Pre-transplantation infectious diseases evaluation
Source: Reprinted from R. Patel and C.V. Paya (1997), with the permission of the American Society for Microbiology

Organs from human immunodeficiency virus (HIV) seropositive prospective donors should not be transplanted, nor should organs from donors who are hepatitis B surface antigen positive. However, it is debatable whether organs from prospective donors who have antibody to the core part of the hepatitis B virus (HBV) should or should not be used, and it has been suggested that organs from donors who have antibody to hepatitis C virus (HCV) should be given only to recipients who have antibody to HCV, and therefore have been exposed to the virus (Patel and Paya, 1997).

Herpesviruses

This family is the main source of viral pathogens in solid-organ and bone-marrow transplant recipients.

There are now eight types of human herpesvirus (HHV), with the clinical spectra of HHV 7 and HHV 8 still to be fully defined. Although we can recover from acute herpesvirus infection, the virus is never eliminated, and each herpesvirus remains in a specific site. For example, herpes simplex virus type one (HSV-1) is latent in the neurons of the trigeminal nerve ganglia. Immunosuppression of transplant patients can result in reactivation of latent infections to produce disease, and it is important to distinguish between primary infections and secondary, or reactivation, infections.

During the first month post-transplantation, HSV is the commonest viral infection (La Rocco, 1997), affecting about 33% of adult transplant recipients and 8% of paediatric transplant recipients (Patel and Paya, 1997). It is usually manifested as labial and oral ulceration, although there may be anogenital or oesophageal involvement. Treatment with aciclovir is usually effective. Prompt laboratory diagnosis of HSV infection can be made by performing the fluorescent antibody test on well-taken vesicle swabs placed in virus transport medium.

CMV has been a major obstacle to successful solid-organ and bone-marrow transplantation, and can lead to increased immunosuppression due to modulation of the immune system, opportunistic infections, organ dysfunction and rejection, and even retransplantation. Economically, the consequences of CMV infection can add 40% to the cost of a transplant (McCarthy et al, 1993). Most cases of CMV disease are not fatal, but morbidity is high. CMV infection typically occurs two to four months after solid-organ transplantation, and up to 100 days in bone-marrow recipients (LaRocco and Burgert, 1997).

There are two main patterns of CMV infection in solid-organ transplant recipients (Falagas and Snydman, 1995):

- Primary infection usually occurs when a CMV-seronegative recipient receives an organ from a CMV-seropositive donor, and these patients are at greatest risk of serious infection. Primary CMV infection occurs in 80% to 100% of seronegative recipients from seropositive donors, and 50% to 70% of these will develop disease.
- Secondary infection due to reactivation or superinfection. Reactivation is usually due to immunosuppression in CMV-seropositive recipients, whereas superinfection usually occurs when a seropositive recipient is infected with CMV from the transplanted organ, the environment or infected blood products. As bone-marrow transplant recipients need more transfusions than solid-organ recipients, they are at greater risk of acquiring CMV disease by this means.

Thus far, ganciclovir is the only available antiviral agent with some degree of efficacy in the prevention of CMV disease. The two main strategies for prevention of CMV disease are:

- prophylaxis, where treatment of all patients begins soon after transplant, and
- pre-emptive, where treatment begins before disease appears, and is given only to those patients at risk of developing disease

Help in defining this risk comes from appropriate diagnostic laboratory tests, whose aim is the rapid and cost-effective detection of clinically significant CMV infection. The polymerase chain reaction (PCR) assay has been shown to be a powerful tool for the early detection of active CMV infection. Refinements in PCR technology allow measurements of the concentration of CMV in plasma (viral load) to be made. This could help determine when ganciclovir treatment begins and enable the therapeutic response to be monitored thereafter (Tong, 1997).

When prophylactic and pre-emptive strategies were compared (Goodrich and Khardori, 1997), it was found that:

- ganciclovir reduces the incidence of CMV disease whether given prophylactically or pre-emptively
- neutropaenia is the main toxic effect of ganciclovir
- only 3% of prophylactically treated patients developed CMV disease, compared with between 13% and 29% of pre-emptively treated patients
- prophylactic therapy is given unnecessarily to patients who do not need it

As with HIV infection, combination therapy has an important role in preventing serious CMV disease. For example, one study involving aciclovir, ganciclovir and CMV hyperimmune globulin examined 77 seronegative recipients who had received organs from seropositive donors. It found that combination therapy reduced the expected disease rate without prophylaxis of between 55% and 60% to 19% (Martin, 1996).

More than 90% of adults have been infected with and therefore harbour EBV. This means that EBV infection in transplant recipients is usually due to reactivation, but may be acquired from the donor organ or blood products (La Rocca, 1997). It seems that simultaneous EBV replication may be one factor that determines whether CMV disease develops. Thus, in a study of renal transplant patients, severe clinical symptoms were seen only in a group among whom both EBV and CMV infections were active (Meyer et al, 1996). Immunosuppression can induce EBV-associated disease ranging from uncomplicated infectious mononucleosis to post-transplantation lymphoproliferative disorder (PTLD), which is most common in the first year after transplantation. The incidence of PTLD varies from 1% for renal transplant recipients to 14% for small-bowel transplant recipients, and treatment with aciclovir and ganciclovir may be useful when given early in the disease (Patel and Paya, 1997). In 1995 EBV was found to be associated with the development of smooth-muscle tumours in three children after liver transplantation (Lee et al, 1995).

Among adult solid-organ transplant recipients, 90% are VZV seropositive and at risk of reactivation resulting in herpes zoster (shingles). This occurs in 5% to 13% of patients about six months after transplantation, and can be treated with aciclovir in addition to VZ immune globulin (Patel and Paya, 1997). The clinical diagnosis of VZV infection can be promptly confirmed by the laboratory, using the direct immunofluorescence test on vesicle swabs or scrapings, or vesicle fluid. Although slow, the culture of herpesviruses from patients undergoing antiviral therapy can be useful in monitoring virus isolates for resistance to antiviral agents.

The involvement of HHV-6 with post-transplantation disease has been more keenly sought in bone-marrow transplant recipients than any other organ transplant population. Various studies have associated HHV-6 activity with skin rash and graft versus host disease, pneumonitis, sinusitis, febrile episodes and bone-marrow suppression. It has been suggested that HHV-6 could be associated with allograft rejection in renal transplant recipients treated with anti-CD3 Mab 9 (OKT3) or antilymphocyte globulin (Braun et al, 1997).

Hepatitis viruses

Infection with HBV and HCV can often cause acute and chronic hepatitis, with substantial morbidity and mortality among transplant recipients undergoing immunosuppression. Primary infection may be acquired from the allograft or by the transfusion of blood products, or there might be a recurrence of pre-existing disease after immunosuppression (La Rocco, 1997). For example, recurrent HBV infection occurs in 80% to 90% of liver transplant patients, with a mortality rate of 50% to 60% (Patel and Paya, 1997).

Papillomaviruses

Solid-organ transplant recipients are at high risk of developing cutaneous and mucosal human papillomavirus (HPV) infection. The degree and length of immunosuppression, and excessive exposure to sunlight are associated with the development of viral warts and skin cancers on sun-exposed sites such as hands, faces and bald heads. Anogenital warts caused by HPVs may be complicated by dysplasia or neoplasia, and there is an increased prevalence of cervical neoplasia in women with renal allografts (Bunney et al, 1992).

Effective treatment against HPV infection is limited. However, interferon therapy combined with laser treatment is a promising option, imiquimod has been released for the treatment of genital warts, and HPV vaccines are at an early stage of development (Gross, 1997).

OTHER VIRUSES

Adenovirus infection may occur in both solid-organ and bone-marrow transplant recipients, and can be acquired by primary infection, reactivation, or by the allograft itself. Among bone-marrow recipients, if infection results in disease, the mortality rate can reach 60% (La Rocco, 1997). Although there have been some reports of successful treatment of adenovirus infection with ribavirin, there are also reports of ribavirin failure (Mann et al, 1998).

About half of all bone-marrow transplantations are complicated by pneumonia. In one centre, respiratory syncytial virus (RSV) accounted for 35% of community-acquired respiratory virus infections, followed by parainfluenza virus (30%), rhinovirus (25%) and influenzavirus (11%); pneumonia often occurred among those infected with RSV (49%) or parainfluenza (22%), but less often among those infected with influenzavirus (<10%) or rhinovirus (3%) (Bowden, 1997). Among solid-organ transplant recipients, the highest incidence of community respiratory viral infections is reported in lung transplant recipients (Wendt, 1997). Whereas the rapid laboratory diagnosis of RSV infection in children relies on the examination of upper respiratory tract specimens, early diagnosis of RSV disease in immunocompromised adults is greatly enhanced by examining bronchoalveolar lavages (Englund et al, 1996).

Enteroviruses seldom cause severe disease after transplantation, but co-infection with CMV may modulate the immune response to produce serious and life-threatening illness (Galama, 1997).

Infection with the fungus *Pneumocystis carinii* is commonly diagnosed in diagnostic virus laboratories, and will be briefly considered here. The laboratory diagnosis of *P. carinii* infection is typically by direct immunofluorescence, and bronchoalveolar lavages are the preferred specimens of choice; induced sputum samples are acceptable, but uninduced sputum samples are not. Prophylactic, low-dose trimethoprim-sulphamethoxazole is effective against *P. carinii* pneumonia among transplant recipients. However, *P. carinii* can cause pneumonia in about 10% of heart, liver, and kidney recipients not receiving prophylaxis during the first six months following transplantation (Patel and Paya, 1997).

Conclusion

After transplantation, the virus laboratory will be involved in the active investigation of infection (or infections) in the patient. In the longer term, when the patient is asymptomatic, the role will become one of surveillance. Because of the latent nature of herpesviruses, it can sometimes be difficult to determine the significance of a positive result in terms of predicting clinical disease. However, progress is being made, especially in the application of PCR techniques to the detection of CMV in the blood.

The increasing use of antiviral therapy means that, in future, the virus laboratory may be undertaking more studies of virus isolates that are resistant to antiviral agents to determine susceptibilities to newer agents. Finally, as xenotransplantation becomes a distant, yet real prospect, we might reasonably expect new virological challenges from unexpected sources.

References

Birchall, M. (1998) Human laryngeal allograft: shift of emphasis in transplantation. *Lancet*; 351: 539–540.

Bowden, R. A. (1997) Respiratory virus infections after marrow transplant: the Fred Hutchinson Cancer Research Center experience. *American Journal of Medicine*; 102 (3A): 27–30.

Braun, D. K., Dominguez, G., Pellett, P. E. (1997) Human herpesvirus 6. *Clinical Microbiology Reviews*; 10: 3, 521–567.

Bunney, M. H., Benton, C., Cubie, H. A. (1992) Warts in the immunodeficient. In: *Viral Warts, Biology and Treatment*. Oxford: Oxford University Press, 2nd edn.

Englund, J. A., Piedra, P. A., Jewell, A. et al (1996) Rapid diagnosis of respiratory syncytial virus infections in immunocompromised adults. *Journal of Clinical Microbiology*; 34: 7, 1649–1653.

Falagas, M. E., Snydman, D. R. (1995) Recurrent cytomegalovirus disease in solid-organ transplant recipients. *Transplantation Proceedings*; 27: 5 (suppl. 1), 34–37.

Galama, J. M. D. (1997) Enteroviral infections in the immunocompromised host. *Reviews in Medical Microbiology*; 8: 1, 33–40.

Goodrich, J., Khardori, N. (1997) Cytomegalovirus: the taming of the beast? *Lancet*; 350: 1718–1719.

Gross, G. (1997) Therapy of human papillomavirus infection and associated epithelial tumors. *Intervirology*; 40: 368–377.

LaRocco, M. T., Burgert, S. J. (1997) Infection in the bone marrow transplant recipient and role of the microbiology laboratory in clinical transplantation. *Clinical Microbiology Reviews*; 10: 2, 277–297.

Lee, E. S., Locker, J., Nalesnik, M. et al (1995) The association of Epstein-Barr virus with smooth-muscle tumors occurring after organ transplantation. *New England Journal of Medicine*; 332: 1, 19–25.

McCarthy, J. M., Karim, M. A., Keown, P. A. (1993) The cost impact of cytomegalovirus disease in renal transplant patients. *Transplantation*; 555: 1277–1282.

Mann, D., Moreb, J., Smith, S., Gian, V. (1998) Failure of intravenous ribavirin in the treatment of invasive adenovirus infection following allogeneic bone marrow transplantation: a case report. *Journal of Infection*; 36: 2, 227–228.

Martin, M. (1996) Combination protocols for prevention of CMV disease in the high risk transplant patient. *Transplantation Proceedings*; 28: 6 (suppl. 2), 12–13.

Meyer, T., Scholz, D., Warnecke, G. et al (1996) Importance of simultaneous active cytomegalovirus and Epstein-Barr virus infection in renal transplantation. *Clinical and Diagnostic Virology*; 6: 79–91.

Patel, R., Paya, C. V. (1997) Infections in solid-organ transplant recipients. *Clinical Microbiology Reviews*; 10: 1, 86–124.

Tong, C. Y. W. (1997) Diagnosis of cytomegalovirus infection and disease. *Journal of Medical Microbiology*; 46: 717–719.

Wendt, C. H. (1997) Community respiratory viruses: organ transplant recipients. *American Journal of Medicine*; 102 (3A): 31–36.

13 HIV and AIDS

A hope beyond the shadow of a dream.

John Keats (1795–1821), *Endymion*.

Over the last 20 years or so, the weight of literature on the acquired immune deficiency syndrome (AIDS) has steadily accumulated as to now pose a serious threat to the sturdiest of library book shelves. Conscious of merely adding to the glut, the largely discursive tone of this chapter is based on the assumption that most healthcare workers (should?) already have a grasp of the basic facts concerning AIDS and its cause. These can be supplemented by reference to a range of reports and journals, which are better equipped than books for prompt dissemination of new information on the subject. For example, the Public Health Laboratory Service and the Scottish Centre for Infection and Environmental Health publish weekly reports and periodic reviews, which present many data on the incidence and prevalence of communicable diseases throughout the UK and Europe. These include up-to-date information and statistical analyses on human immunodeficiency virus (HIV) infection and AIDS in these regions.

In the United States the Centers for Disease Control, Atlanta, publish *The Morbidity and Mortality Weekly Report*, which was to become the harbinger of the AIDS epidemic when, in 1981, it reported an increasing number of young homosexual men with the previously rare *Pneumocystis carinii* pneumonia (CDC, 1981). In 1982, as more 'opportunistic' infections and cancers such as Kaposi's sarcoma were found in this group, these conditions helped establish a definition of AIDS. Haemophiliacs, blood transfusion recipients and injecting drug users were also succumbing to AIDS, and by 1983 the causative agent, HIV, was discovered. In that year only 15 cases of AIDS were reported in the UK; by the end of 1996, over 13,700 cases of AIDS had been reported in the UK, and worldwide at least eight million cases of AIDS and about 30 million HIV infections (*CDR Review*, 1997), making HIV one of the top 10 causes of death in the world.

Despite advances in drug therapy, the outlook for many HIV-infected individuals remains bleak, and skilled, sensitive nursing care can help to ameliorate the fears of these patients. Similarly, much can be done to allay the anxieties of those undertaking HIV testing for the first time. It is important to note that blood specimens should be collected from the patient, after counselling, during the appointment and that blood specimens brought by the patient should be treated with suspicion. The collection of blood is discussed in Chapter 3, but it is worth emphasising that HIV/AIDS patients must be carefully managed because their blood is infectious.

HIV is a ribonucleic acid (RNA) virus belonging to the *Retroviridae* family, whose unique mode of replication is described briefly in Chapter 2. There are two types of HIV: HIV-1 is found throughout the world, whereas HIV-2 is largely restricted to West Africa. There are at least six subtypes (A F), or *clades,* of HIV-1. Clade B is the predominant subtype in the Americas and Europe, clades B, C and E are associated with the Asian epidemic, and clades A, C and D are most often found in Africa (Levy, 1996). Knowledge of subtypes is important in determining the relative virulence of certain subtypes, in studying resistance to antiretroviral drugs, and in planning future vaccination strategies.

Of the estimated three million new HIV infections each year, at least 95% are in the developing world (Davison and Nicoll, 1997), where an important factor in the spread of HIV has been the migration of poor, sexually active individuals from rural to urban settings. For example, in sub-Saharan Africa between 1960 and 1980, more than 75 military coups occurred in 30 countries, and the number of urban centres with more than 500,000 people rose from three to 28 (Quinn, 1995). Such massive migration combined with poor medical services, social disruption and epidemics of sexually transmitted diseases probably contributed to the spread of HIV. Tourism and the drug trade have lent an international dimension to increase global dissemination further.

A striking feature in the evolution of the AIDS pandemic has been its facility to affect new populations. For example, what began as a disease of young, white, male homosexuals has developed so that in the United States and Europe most AIDS cases are among men who have sex with men and among injecting drug users, whereas in Africa and Asia AIDS is mainly spread heterosexually. Different modes of HIV transmission can predominate in different areas of the same country. For instance, in the UK more than 70% of reported AIDS cases acquired HIV infection through sexual intercourse between men; most of these cases were reported from London and the south-east of England (Macdonald, 1997). Similarly, most heterosexual transmission in the UK has been reported from the Thames regions (McGarrigle et al, 1997). In contrast, by the end of 1996 35% of AIDS cases due to injecting drug use diagnosed in the UK were reported in Scotland (Hughes, 1997). However, the number of reported HIV infections in Scotland associated with injecting drug use has fallen from a peak reached in 1986 (Robertson et al, 1986), with successful needle-exchange and health education programmes probably contributing to this fall (Madden et al, 1997).

In the UK further limited grounds for cautious optimism came in June 1998, when a report issued before the 12th World AIDS Conference suggested that HIV prevention in the UK had been more successful than in most western European countries (Joint United Nations Programme on HIV/AIDS, 1998). However, two points help to illustrate the importance of maintaining a global awareness of the disease. First, most cases of paediatric HIV infection in the UK have occurred in the London area: by the end of January 1997, of the 298 cases of mother-to-child transmission reported there, 79% occurred mostly in black Africans, who were presumed to have acquired their infections through heterosexual exposure abroad (Molesworth and Tookey, 1997). Second, heterosexual transmission of HIV in the UK has continued, although data to the end of 1996 showed that three-quarters of these cases were associated with infection abroad (McGarrigle et al, 1997).

Concern about occupational exposure of healthcare workers to HIV in the UK has been addressed, and studies have shown that there is no evidence of risk if HIV-infected blood is in contact with intact skin. The average risk for HIV transmission after a percutaneous exposure to HIV-infected blood is about 0.3%, whereas the risk of acquiring HIV through mucous membrane exposure is 0.09%. These risks can be further reduced if antiretroviral prophylaxis is taken as soon as possible after occupational exposure. The UK Health Departments recommend 'that every NHS Trust or other health care setting should develop a post exposure policy and a protocol' (UK Health Departments, 1997).

By the end of the 1980s it was clear that HIV infection could be transmitted through blood transfusion and blood product treatment. Throughout the industrialised world, claims for compensation, civil litigation, public inquiries and criminal charges against high-ranking health officials served to emphasise the point that the value of preventive medicine is only recognised through its failures. Since October 1985 all blood and plasma donations in the UK have been screened for HIV antibody. Between then and the end of 1996, two HIV-infected blood donations were accepted for transfusion; each donation had been made during the 'window' period between infection and the development of HIV antibody (Mortimer and Spooner, 1997). In the UK the main recipients of blood products are congenital haemophiliacs, who are deficient in clotting factor. Since 1983, when the first AIDS cases were reported in association with the treatment of haemophilia, more than 1,200 haemophiliacs in the UK have been infected (Mortimer and Spooner, 1997). The use of blood products which have been heat-treated has virtually eliminated the risk of HIV infection from this source.

Rapid progress against HIV infection has been made in chemotherapy and combination drug therapy is now commonplace in the developed world; indeed, the hypothesis has been advanced that a seven-drug combination of currently available antiretroviral agents could cure or control HIV/AIDS (Collins and Sakamoto, 1997). It is unsurprising therefore that the pharmaceutical industry gives relatively scant regard to high-volume/low-profit items like vaccines, favouring instead low-volume/high-profit items such as therapeutic drugs. Nevertheless, to prevent further infections worldwide a vaccine is needed, and there is a tension between this need and the existing poor financial incentives to develop one. The little work which is currently being done on HIV vaccines is firmly based in molecular technology. Some workers question this strategy, arguing in favour of a traditional approach to vaccine development, and remain unimpressed with what they see as a general lack of enthusiasm and commitment to a vaccination programme (Oxford et al, 1998).

J. G. Ballard had retroviruses in mind when, in 1992, he wrote: 'The greater the advances of modern medicine, the more urgent our need for diseases we cannot understand' (Ballard, 1996).

Since our need, as he expressed it, was met in 1981, our understanding of HIV and AIDS has been much enriched, and our aim must be to ensure that the knowledge gained by HIV/AIDS research is used to help people everywhere. But to assume that a global cure for, or control of, HIV/AIDS can be achieved by simply applying this expanding fund of biomedical knowledge to the problem is to evince dangerous optimism. The bulk of biomedical research is undertaken in the industrialised countries, where the global research agenda is set, and is chiefly aimed at expanding fundamental knowledge of HIV/AIDS. Under increasing media scrutiny, researchers have sought to justify a 'back-to-basic science' approach by pointing to the pursuit of truth; an essential widening of the knowledge base as a prerequisite to further advancement. However, these arguments fail to impress those millions of individuals worldwide, infected with or affected by HIV, who have an impatience with the scientific process and who understandably wish for (or demand) a more clinical approach with greater emphasis on treatment.

The pursuit of pure knowledge requires talent; applying it properly needs intellect. One challenge for researchers in the developed world is to accept their responsibility to ensure that the fruits of their research may soon be harvested in the developing world. A tall order indeed, because a means must be found of marshalling the modest global expenditure on HIV/AIDS prevention, care and research, and of addressing the disparity existing between rich and poor countries. Clearly, HIV is not an equal opportunity disease (Fig 13.1).

The Global AIDS Strategy was launched in 1986, funded by official development assistance (ODA) from industrialised donor countries. International funding for AIDS research, treatment and care rose from under $1 million in that year to $212 million in 1990. However, whereas ODA funding to AIDS saw a rate of increase of 127% between 1987 and 1988, this fell to between 4% and 11% between 1990 and 1993 (Laws, 1996). The very real phenomenon of donor fatigue syndrome was at work in Paris in 1994 when the Heads of Governments Summit on AIDS convened to muster financial support for the Global AIDS Strategy; the expected funds did not transpire. Donor fatigue is partly induced by competing demands from disparate and desperate sources, be they national AIDS programmes or agencies involved in humanitarian ventures as a result of natural disasters or ethnic conflict. A perceived lack of success of certain funding projects, combined with poor administrative coordination, also contribute to an air of general frustration (Laws, 1996).

The various strands currently engaged in understanding and preventing further development of the pandemic have to address a range of individual and societal issues. Drawing these into a cohesive global

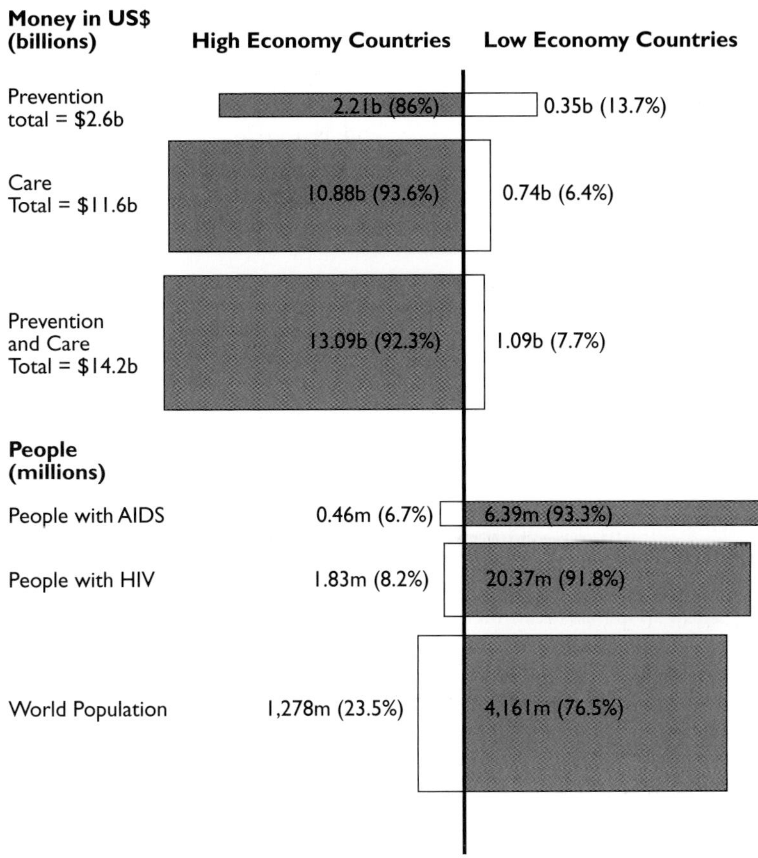

Fig 13.1 People with HIV/AIDS and the cost of HIV/AIDS prevention and care in high- and low-economy countries: the world disparity, *c.*1993
Source: Reprinted from J. Broomberg (1996) with the author's permission

strategy is a task requiring an ability to recognise that change is possible. But the price of recognition depends on our realising that because some concepts may be difficult to grasp, it should not stop us reaching for them. For example, let us consider HIV epidemiology and human rights. A risk-reduction approach that advises men and women to reduce their number of sexual partners carries less weight in areas where the risk to married, and unmarried, women is largely determined by the sexual behaviour of their male partners, who may invoke the threat of physical violence or divorce to ensure compliance of HIV-aware women in unprotected sexual relationships. The subordinate status of many women worldwide is central to the solution of the problem of HIV infection in this group, and requires the recognition and promotion of a human rights dimension if appropriate preventive strategies are to be devised. Similar consideration should be given to human rights issues in relation to HIV prevention among threatened or persecuted groups of gay men, lesbians, injecting drug misusers, and other 'minority' populations.

One of the difficulties with this approach is that there is a sense in which HIV/AIDS is a public health problem, which it is; but ominously entwined is a sense in which HIV/AIDS is the 'property' of medical science, which it is not. Just as medical scientists may construe human rights concerns as meddling in a problem of epidemiology, they, in turn, can be reminded of their obligation to understand their work in its proper social and global context.

As our understanding of HIV/AIDS becomes more sophisticated, our aim remains simple: the cure or control of HIV/AIDS. In focusing our aim as the pandemic evolves and changes, we similarly must be prepared to evolve and refine strategies. Perhaps the true test of our sophistication would be to achieve simplicity through refinement.

References

Ballard, J. G. (1996) *A User's Guide to the Millennium*. London: HarperCollins, p. 297.

Broomberg, J. (1996) Global spending on HIV/AIDS prevention, care, and research. In: Mann, J., Tarantola, D. (eds) *AIDS in the World II*. New York: Oxford University Press.

CDC (1981) Pneumocystis pneumonia – Los Angeles. *Morbidity and Mortality Weekly Report*; 30: 250–252.

CDR Review (1997) The epidemiology of HIV infection and AIDS; 7: 9, R118–R136.

Collins, D. O., Sakamoto, A. (1997) Cure or control of HIV/AIDS? *Medical Hypotheses*; 48: 489–490.

Davison, K., Nicoll, A. (1997) The changing global epidemiology of HIV infection and AIDS. *CDR Review*; 7: 9, R134–R136.

Hughes, G. (1997) An overview of the HIV and AIDS epidemic in the United Kingdom. *CDR Review*; 7: 9, R121–R122.

Joint United Nations Programme on HIV/AIDS and the World Health Organisation (WHO) (1998) *Report on the Global HIV/AIDS Epidemic 9 June 1998*. Geneva: UNAIDS/WHO.

Laws, M. (1996) International funding of the global AIDS Strategy: official development assistance. In: Mann, J., Tarantola, D. (eds) *AIDS in the World II*. New York: Oxford University Press.

Levy, J. A. (1996) HIV heterogeneity in transmission and pathogenesis. In: Mann, J., Tarantola, D. (eds) *AIDS in the World II*. New York: Oxford University Press.

Macdonald, N. D. (1997) AIDS and HIV infection acquired through sexual intercourse between men. *CDR Review*; 7: 9, R123–R124.

McGarrigle, C., Gilbart, V., Nicoll, A. (1997) AIDS and HIV infection acquired heterosexually. *CDR Review*; 7: 9, R125–R128.

Madden, P. B., Lamagni, T., Hope, V. et al (1997) The HIV epidemic in injecting drug users. *CDR Review*; 7: 9, R128–R130.

Molesworth, A., Tookey, P. (1997) Paediatric AIDS and HIV infection. *CDR Review*; 7: 9, R132–R134.

Mortimer, J. Y., Spooner, R. J. D. (1997) HIV infection transmitted through blood product treatment, blood transfusion, and tissue transplantation. *CDR Review*; 7: 9, R130–R132.

Oxford, J. S., Addawe, M., Lambkin, R. (1998) AIDS vaccine development: let a thousand flowers bloom. *Journal of Clinical Pathology*; 51: 725–730.

Quinn, T. C. (1995) Population migration and the spread of types 1 and 2 human immunodeficiency viruses. In: Roizman, B. (ed) *Infectious Diseases in an Age of Change*. Washington: National Academy of Sciences.

Robertson, J. R., Bucknall, A. B. V., Welsby, P. D. et al (1986) Epidemic of AIDS related virus (HTLV-III/LAV) infection among intravenous drug abusers. *British Medical Journal*; 292: 527–529.

UK Health Departments (June 1997) *Guidelines on Post-exposure Prophylaxis for Health Care Workers Occupationally Exposed to HIV.* London: Department of Health.

14 Antiviral therapy

The desire to take medicine is perhaps the greatest feature which distinguishes man from animals.

Sir William Osler (1849–1919).

In 1909 Paul Ehrlich cured a rabbit of syphilis by injecting it with a compound called Salvarsan, which he synthesised in his laboratory. For Ehrlich, a hard-drinking eccentric with a Groucho Marx cigar and a complete disregard for laboratory protocol (De Kruif, 1927), this justified his contention that 'we must learn to shoot the microbes with magic bullets', and he has since become known as the founding father of chemotherapy. The advent of antibiotics soon followed, and many bacterial targets were sought and successfully hit by arsenals of newly developed magic bullets such as penicillin and streptomycin.

Meanwhile, antiviral therapy lagged far behind. One reason is that viruses were discovered much later than other microbes. Another reason is that the intimate association of virus and cell was thought to preclude effective chemotherapy; it seemed that in order to attack the virus, the host cell would sustain too much damage. The small advances in antiviral therapy therefore came from chance discoveries of the beneficial effects of compounds intended for use in other conditions. For example, in the early 1950s, thiosemicarbazones, which had originally been used for the treatment of tuberculosis, were shown to be potent inhibitors of poxvirus replication, and in 1963 a derivative, Marboran, was found to be effective in the prophylaxis of smallpox infection. Idoxuridine, an anti-herpes compound, was originally synthesised in 1959 as an anti-cancer drug, and was shown to be effective against herpes keratoconjunctivitis.

However, with the realisation that there are certain events in the virus replication cycle which are unique and virus specific, the idea arose that these events represented possible targets for selective antiviral therapy, aimed at virus-infected cells. The revolution in antiviral therapy began in 1977 with the launch of acyclovir (now aciclovir) as Zovirax, a safe, specific, anti-herpes agent. By its mode of action, targeting a particular point of the virus replication cycle, aciclovir became the paradigm antiviral therapy. The main advances in antiviral therapy have occurred with herpesviruses, hepatitis viruses, human immunodeficiency viruses (HIV) and respiratory viruses. Progress has been such that a working party was recently established to review problems specific to the development and evaluation of antiviral agents in man (Working Party of the BSAC/SPM, 1997).

Herpesviruses

Aciclovir is a nucleoside analogue. In Chapter 2 nucleic acid replication was considered, and we noted that the four basic building blocks of deoxyribonucleic acid (DNA) are adenine, cytosine, thymine and guanine. In its active form aciclovir resembles deoxyguanosine triphosphate, which contains guanine and becomes incorporated into the virus DNA, but because it is an 'abnormal' molecule, it disrupts the growing chain of viral DNA and replication stops. There are three stages. First, aciclovir is selectively taken into herpes-infected cells. Second, it is 'activated' by the herpes-specific enzyme, thymidine kinase; it is this virus-specific enzyme which gives aciclovir its exquisite specificity. Third, 'activated' aciclovir stops herpesvirus replication (Fig 14.1).

Aciclovir is available worldwide for intravenous, oral and topical use, and is the treatment of choice for severe herpes simplex virus (HSV) and varicella zoster virus (VZV) infections in immunocompetent and immunocompromised patients. For example, in HSV infection of the neonatal central nervous system (CNS), aciclovir treatment has reduced the mortality rate from 90% in untreated cases to 12% (Wutzler, 1997). Similarly, aciclovir treatment has reduced the mortality rate from HSV encephalitis from 70% in untreated cases to about 25%. However, there is a need for antiviral drugs which have greater CNS penetration.

Stage 1

Selective entry of Zovirax into herpes-infected cells

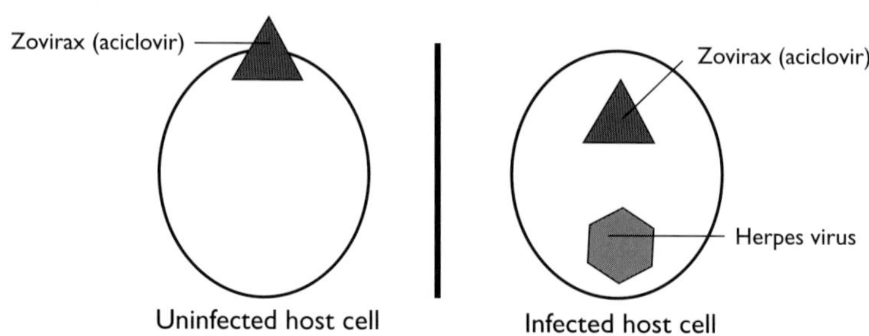

Zovirax enters herpes virus-infected cells much more readily than uninfected cells. This is probably because Zovirax needs a diffusion gradient to cross the cell membrane. Because Zovirax is not activated within uninfected cells, it is not removed. Therefore, the concentration of Zovirax builds up quickly inside the cell membrane and prevents the entry of more drug into these uninfected cells. When activated, Zovirax as such is removed, which allows more to cross the membrane and take its place.

Stage 2

Phosphorylation of Zovirax to the 'active' form, aciclovir triphosphate

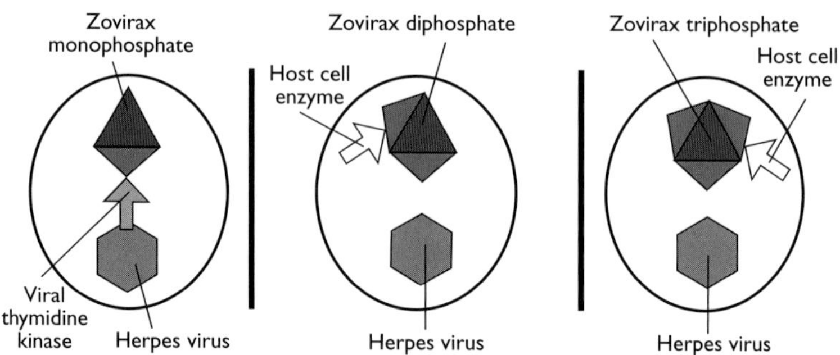

Before Zovirax can exert antiviral activity, it must eventually be converted to aciclovir triphosphate, the molecule that interferes with viral DNA replication. The first step in activation is that aciclovir is converted to the monophosphate by a herpes-specific thymidine kinase enzyme. It is this herpes virus-specific activation that makes Zovirax unique. Host cell enzymes assist the addition of a second and third phosphate group, to form aciclovir diphosphate and aciclovir triphosphate.

Stage 3

Inhibition of herpes virus multiplication by aciclovir triphosphate

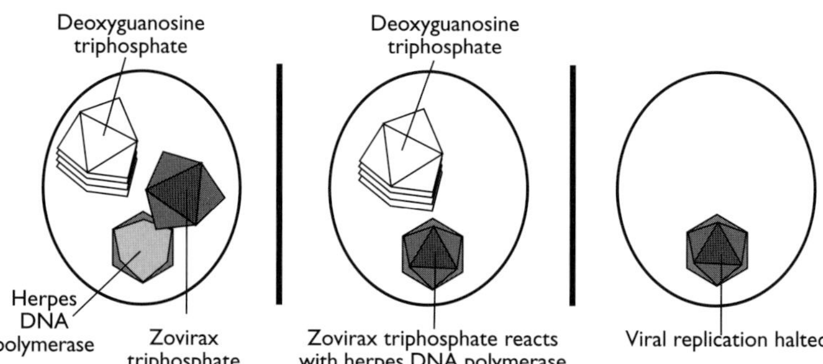

Multiplication of herpes viruses depends on continuing replication of viral DNA. A key component is deoxyguanosine triphosphate which provides the guanine base incorporated into viral DNA.

Activated Zovirax, as the triphosphate, resembles deoxyguanosine triphosphate closely enough to compete as a substrate for viral DNA polymerase, the enzyme that assists incorporation into DNA. Zovirax triphosphate is not a good substrate for host cell DNA polymerase, and hence does not compete to any significant degree for incorporation into host DNA.

Once Zovirax is included, the viral DNA chain becomes 'abnormal': It can add no further building units, and the chain terminates, halting viral replication.

Fig 14.1 Mode of action of Zovirax (aciclovir)

Source: Reprinted with permission of Glaxo Wellcome plc, Greenford, Middlesex UB6 ONN

A limitation of nucleoside analogues, such as aciclovir, is that the bioavailability following oral administration is only around 15% to 30%. This problem has been addressed by giving a 'prodrug' which is converted *in vivo* to the active form. For instance, after oral administration of the prodrug valaciclovir, it is quickly metabolised to aciclovir. Similarly, famciclovir is the prodrug of penciclovir, which has a similar anti-herpesvirus spectrum to aciclovir.

Fortunately, aciclovir-resistant strains of HSV and VZV do not present a serious clinical problem in immunocompetent patients, with less than 3% of clinical isolates yielding resistant strains (Field and Whitley, 1998). Aciclovir-resistant strains of HSV are most often encountered among immunocompromised patients, of whom around 5% may shed resistant virus. The most common cause of resistance is the presence of virus lacking the thymidine kinase enzyme, in whose absence aciclovir is ineffective. Foscarnet acts by inhibiting DNA polymerase, and is active against thymidine kinase-deficient strains of HSV and VZ, although it is relatively toxic.

Cytomegalovirus (CMV) is an important pathogen as it commonly infects transplant patients and is the most common life-threatening viral infection in HIV-infected patients. In the last 10 years three drugs have enabled progress to be made in the treatment of CMV disease: ganciclovir, foscarnet and cidofovir are inhibitors of CMV DNA polymerase. Although effective, their toxicity requires careful patient monitoring. Ganciclovir has a similar mode of action to aciclovir but better anti-CMV activity, although ganciclovir is more toxic and virus-encoded kinase-deficient mutants can arise. Whereas ganciclovir can be given intravenously or orally, foscarnet is usually given intravenously as it is poorly absorbed after oral administration. In addition, foscarnet is more toxic than ganciclovir, causing side-effects such as nephrotoxicity and electrolyte imbalances (Vogel et al, 1997).

Cidofovir is a broad-spectrum anti-DNA virus agent active against all herpesviruses (including Epstein-Barr Virus-associated diseases such as hairy leukoplakia), papovaviruses, adenoviruses and poxviruses, but is used primarily as an anti-CMV agent (De Clercq, 1997), where it has been effective in the treatment of CMV retinitis when ganciclovir and/or foscarnet have failed (Ives, 1997). It is one of a new series of so-called acyclic nucleoside phosphonates that achieve their antiviral effect by having a greater affinity for virus DNA polymerase than cellular DNA polymerase (De Clercq, 1998). An advantage of these drugs is that their prolonged antiviral action requires fewer doses, and thus encourages better patient compliance.

Hepatitis viruses

Hepatitis A virus and hepatitis E virus cause acute disease, and are not particularly severe infections. However, hepatitis B (HBV), hepatitis C (HCV) and hepatitis D (HDV) may cause chronic infections with serious liver disease, and hence research has been directed towards antiviral therapy for chronic infections caused by these viruses. As HDV is dependent on the presence of HBV, investigations into appropriate treatments have concentrated on HBV and HCV.

In hepatitis B, the aim of antiviral therapy is either the prevention of persistent HBV replication at high concentrations, or the enhancement of the immune response to HBV, or both. The interferons are a family of glycoproteins with a broad antiviral action which are produced naturally by the host at an early stage during viral infection. They are very potent, can modulate the immune response, and can be used in the treatment of malignant disease (Toy, 1983). At present, treatment of chronic HBV infection with injected alpha interferon is the only approved therapy and it can have potentially severe side-effects. Among patients with HBV e antigen (HBeAg) positive chronic hepatitis B, the loss of HBeAg is associated with improved survival. However, there is debate about the efficacy of interferon therapy, especially among patients of Asian origin, and the question has been asked whether interferon therapy leads to loss of HBeAg or merely hastens spontaneous conversion among those already destined to do so (Carithers, 1998).

Encouraging results have been achieved with oral lamivudine, a nucleoside analogue which suppresses viral replication (Jaeckel and Manns, 1997; Lai et al, 1998). However, lamivudine does not eliminate HBV, and the development of resistant strains is a significant clinical problem.

Before HCV was identified as the main cause of non-A, non-B hepatitis, alpha interferon had shown limited benefit, yet became licensed for treatment. The high cost of interferon and its relatively low efficacy have given rise to concerns about the appropriateness of interferon monotherapy (Terrault and Wright, 1995). Ribavirin is a nucleoside analogue of guanosine with a broad spectrum of activity against RNA and DNA viruses, and has been used in treating HCV infection. However, when ribavirin was used in combination with interferon, one study found that viral clearance rates among patients a year after discontinuation of treatment were 42% for combination therapy, compared with 20% for interferon alone (Reichard et al, 1998). Further clinical trials are in progress, and perhaps experience gained in the use of combination therapy for tuberculosis and HIV infection could be usefully applied to the treatment of chronic hepatitis infections.

HIVs

Although there is an average of 10 to 12 years of clinical latency, HIV is actively replicating in most patients, producing up to a billion new viruses each day, with a half-life of around six hours in plasma. At present, antiretroviral therapy aims to reduce the viral load below the detection limits of currently available laboratory assays. Before considering strategy, let us look at some antiretroviral drugs.

The main drugs in use are reverse transcriptase inhibitors and protease inhibitors. Reverse transcriptase (RT) is an enzyme found in HIV which mediates the production of viral DNA from viral ribonucleic acid (RNA), and is targeted by two types of drug: nucleoside RT inhibitors (NRTI) and non-nucleoside RT inhibitors (NNRTI). Zidovudine, or azidothymidine (AZT), originally developed as an anti-cancer agent, was the first widely prescribed NRTI. It is an analogue of thymidine, and its uptake prevents further viral DNA synthesis. By the end of the 1980s HIV treatment consisted of zidovudine monotherapy. If this failed, the NRTIs didanosine and/or zalcitabine were used in combination with zidovudine, often with improved results. A more recent and potent NRTI, abacavir, shows especially good penetration of the CNS (Schmit and Weber, 1997). Nevirapine, delavirdine and loviride are NNRTIs which are chemically heterogeneous, but share the property of inhibiting RT and are therefore available to augment further multiple choices of combination therapy.

During the replication cycle of HIV type 1, a protein called Gag-Pol is produced. An enzyme called a protease splits this protein into virus core proteins and other enzymes. If the protease is inactivated, non-infectious viruses are produced. Saquinavir was the first protease inhibitor to be described, and others include ritonavir, indinavir and nelfinavir.

From zidovudine monotherapy of the 1980s, the current therapeutic approach is triple-drug combination therapy (Gazzard and Moyle, 1998), with the aim of an early and aggressive assault on the virus, mainly to counteract variants (Ho, 1995). HIV has a high level of replication and a high mutation rate, producing many variants. Therefore a combination of drugs which could 'knock out' more variants would be more effective than monotherapy. In addition, at an early stage of infection there are fewer variants in the virus population compared with chronic infection; as viral resistance is the main reason for treatment failure, the more homogeneous the virus population is, the greater the chance of successful therapy at an early stage. Finally, the availability of even more potent drugs would augment those drugs presently in use.

However, the early, aggressive, highly active antiretroviral therapy approach is not favoured by all (Levy, 1998), and concerns over toxicity, and the limiting of future options, have been raised, suggesting a need to place more emphasis on activating the immune system.

Respiratory viruses

Influenza epidemics can cause severe morbidity, mortality and economic loss worldwide, and the availability of an effective vaccine has undoubted benefits for the control of influenza in human populations (Nichol et al, 1995). However, the rate of vaccination in high-risk groups is poor, ranging from 4.5% to 19.5% (Wiselka, 1994), in which case antiviral prophylaxis or treatment would be appropriate.

Amantadine, whose antiviral activity was first described in 1964, is the only anti-influenza drug licensed in the UK. Along with its analogue, rimantadine, it is effective against influenzavirus A, but not influenzaviruses B or C, and acts by inhibiting the uncoating of infecting virus. During influenza outbreaks, amantadine can be used prophylactically for:

- unvaccinated individuals at high risk and unvaccinated healthcare workers
- those for whom vaccination is contraindicated, or of limited use because of immunodeficiency
- supplementing vaccinated individuals at high risk
- augmenting the protection already conferred by vaccination of nursing-home residents and staff (Wiselka, 1994)

Treatment with amantadine not only reduces the severity of influenzal symptoms, but may reduce spread (Couch et al, 1986). Although amantadine-resistant viruses have been found, amantadine therapy still remains effective (Oxford, 1995). Zanamivir is a neuraminidase inhibitor which is effective against both influenza A and influenza B, and could have a future role in the control of influenza. However, influenza B causes only about 35% of cases, and zanamivir has the disadvantage of requiring aerosol administration to the respiratory tract (Couch, 1997).

Since its discovery in 1972, ribavirin has been demonstrated to show activity against a range of DNA and RNA viruses. Aerosolised ribavirin treatment has been effective against acute influenza A and influenza B infections in young adults, and has been especially widely used against respiratory syncytial virus infection in infants and young children (Fernandez et al, 1986). It is interesting to note that ribavirin-resistant mutants are rare, possibly because the agent acts on several different targets, or perhaps because of as yet undefined cellular effects (Field and Whitley, 1998).

Progress in X-ray crystallography has allowed researchers to acquire detailed knowledge of enzyme structure, enabling potential targets for antiviral attack to be precisely defined. For example, neuraminidase is an enzyme that appears on the surface of the influenza virus in the form of a spike; it is involved in the release and spread of virus from infected cells. Encouraging results have been obtained with the extravagantly named Neu5Ac2en, which interferes with the action of neuraminidase (Oxford, 1995), and we might anticipate the development of this strategy towards more 'tailor-made' antivirals rather than reliance on the empirical try-it-and-see approach, which characterised early developments in antiviral therapy.

Although rhinovirus infections are generally mild, they can also have serious outcomes (Stenhouse, 1967; McMillan et al, 1993). As we delve further into what Ballard has called the 'microverse' (Ballard, 1996), it seems that a cure for the common cold may be found by applying molecular biological techniques to study the anatomy of the rhinovirus/cell-receptor relationship. Already there are compounds such as enviroxime, which fills the receptor 'pocket' and blocks rhinovirus attachment, and pirodavir, which inhibits viral replication. First-generation antihistamine treatment is likely to play an important role in the alleviation of common cold symptoms if not exerting a specific antiviral effect; clemastine fumarate has been approved for non-prescription use in the USA, and in a recent study brompheniramine maleate was shown to be effective in the treatment of the sneezing, runny nose and cough associated with rhinovirus colds (Gwaltney and Druce, 1997).

The problems of viral resistance and antiviral toxicity present the main challenges for the future, and the application of combination therapy to the treatment of viral infections is likely to prove more valuable than monotherapy. Meanwhile, it seems that our exploration of the 'microverse' will yield many exciting theoretical possibilities for treatment, whose practical applications will remain to be determined.

References

Ballard, J. G. (1996) *A User's Guide to the Millennium*. London: HarperCollins, p. 278.

Carithers, R. L. (1998) Effect of interferon on hepatitis B. *Lancet*; 351: 157.

Couch, R.B., Kasel, J. A., Glezen, W. P. et al (1986) Influenza: its control in persons and populations. *Journal of Infectious Diseases*; 153: 3, 431–440.

Couch, R. B. (1997) A new antiviral agent for influenza – is there a clinical niche? *New England Journal of Medicine*; 337: 13, 927–928.

De Clercq, E. (1997) In search of a selective antiviral chemotherapy. *Clinical Microbiology Reviews*; 10: 4, 674–693.

De Clercq, E. (1998) Acyclic nucleoside phosphonates: a new dimension to the chemotherapy of DNA virus and retrovirus infections. *Journal of Medical Microbiology*; 47: 1–3.

De Kruif, P., Ehrlich, P. (1927) *Microbe Hunters*. London: Jonathan Cape.

Fernandez, H., Banks, C., Smith, R. (1986) Ribavirin: a clinical overview. *European Journal of Epidemiology*; 2: 1, 1–14.

Field, H. J., Whitley, R. J. (1998) Antiviral chemotherapy. In: Mahy, B. W. J., Collier, L. (eds) *Topley and Wilson's Microbiology and Microbial Infections*, vol. 1: *Virology*. London: Arnold.

Gazzard, B., Moyle, G. on behalf of the British HIV Association Writing Committee (1998) Consensus statement: 1998 revision to the British HIV Association guidelines for antiretroviral treatment of HIV seropositive individuals. *Lancet*; 352: 314–316.

Gwaltney, J. M., Druce, H. M. (1997) Efficacy of brompneniramine maleate for the treatment of rhinovirus colds. *Clinical Infectious Diseases*; 25: 1188–1194.

Ho, D. D. (1995) Time to hit HIV, early and hard. *New England Journal of Medicine*; 333: 7, 450–451.

Ives, D. I. (1997) Cytomegalovirus disease in AIDS. *AIDS*; 11: 1791–1797.

Jaeckel, E., Manns, M. P. (1997) Experience with lamivudine against hepatitis B virus. *Intervirology*; 40: 322–336.

Lai Ching-Lung, Chien Rong-Nan, Leung, N.W.Y. et al (1998) A one-year trial of lamivudine for chronic hepatitis B. *New England Journal of Medicine*; 339: 2, 61–68.

Levy, J. A. (1998) Caution: should we be treating HIV infection early? *Lancet*; 352: 982–983.

McMillan, J. A., Weiner, L. B., Higgins, A. M., Macknight, K. (1993) Rhinovirus infection associated with serious illness among pediatric patients. *Pediatric Infectious Disease Journal*; 12: 4, 321–325.

Nichol, K. L., Lind, A., Margolis, K. L. et al (1995) The effectiveness of vaccination against influenza in healthy, working adults. *New England Journal of Medicine*; 333: 14, 889–893.

Oxford, J. S. (1995) Quo vadis antiviral agents for herpes, influenza and HIV? *Journal of Medical Microbiology*; 43: 1–3.

Reichard, O., Norkrans, G., Fryden, A. (1998) Randomised, double-blind, placebo-controlled trial of interferon alpha-2b with and without ribavirin for chronic hepatitis C. *Lancet*; 351: 83–87.

Report of a Working Party of the British Society for Antimicrobial Chemotherapy and the Society of Pharmaceutical Medicine (1997) The clinical evaluation of antiviral agents. *Journal of Antimicrobial Chemotherapy*; 40: suppl. B, 1–67.

Schmit, J., Weber, B. (1997) Recent advances in antiretroviral therapy and HIV infection monitoring. *Intervirology*; 40: 304–321.

Stenhouse, A. C. (1967) Rhinovirus infection in acute exacerbations of chronic bronchitis: a controlled prospective study. *British Medical Journal*; 3: 461–463.

Terrault, N., Wright, T. (1995) Interferon and hepatitis C. *New England Journal of Medicine*; 332: 1509–1511.

Toy, J. L. (1983) The interferons. *Clinical and Experimental Immunology*; 54: 1–13.

Vogel, J., Scholz, M., Cinatl, J. (1997) Treatment of cytomegalovirus diseases. *Intervirology*; 40: 357–367.

Wiselka, M. (1994) Influenza: diagnosis, management, and prophylaxis. *British Medical Journal*; 308: 1341–1345.

Wutzler, P. (1997) Antiviral therapy of herpes simplex and varicella-zoster virus infections. *Intervirology*; 40: 343–356.

15 Oncogenic viruses

Entities should not be multiplied beyond necessity.

Attributed to William of Ockham (1300–1348), *Quodlibeta Septem.*

Rabies, Ebola, Lassa fever, poliomyelitis: each name evokes an image of relentless cellular destruction by viruses, resulting in serious illness or death. However, this widespread view of the virus as an aggressive cellular vandal is only part of the truth about the virus/cell relationship, because it ignores the intimate association which can occur between virus and cell.

An alternative to cellular destruction is one whereby viral nucleic acid becomes integrated into host deoxyribonucleic acid (DNA). It is the nature of this relationship which determines, to a large extent, whether previously normal cells are transformed into tumour cells. The development of ideas linking viruses to cancer began in the early 1900s.

In 1908 Ellerman and Bang showed that seemingly spontaneous chicken leukaemias could be transmitted to other chickens by means of cell-free filtrates. In 1911 Peyton Rous discovered that a chicken sarcoma, a solid tumour, was caused by a virus, later called Rous sarcoma virus (RSV). Initially regarded as laboratory curiosities by cancer researchers, it became apparent over the next 50 years that more animal tumours could be induced by viruses. Indeed, minds were concentrated when it was shown that some human adenoviruses could induce tumours in rats, mice and hamsters.

How could tumour viruses transform normal cells into cancerous cells? In the 1920s work with bacteriophages, that is viruses which infect bacteria, had shown that virus nucleic acid could become permanently integrated into bacterial nucleic acid. Might it be that viral genes became integrated into animal chromosomal DNA and passed from one generation to another, to become 'switched on' by some environmental influence? In the early 1960s Robert Huebner and George Todaro proposed the concept of the *oncogene*, or cancer gene. This was founded on the discovery that particular viral genes influenced certain retroviruses to form tumours. However, by the mid-1970s it was recognised that the oncogenes carried by some cancer-causing viruses were not true viral genes. The oncogenes, which had previously been involved in cell growth and multiplication, had simply been 'stolen' by viruses from the DNA of the host cells they had infected and were subsequently altered (Krontiris, 1995).

The idea that viral nucleic acid became integrated into host DNA made sense, considering that most animal oncogenic viruses contained DNA. However, viruses such as RSV contained ribonucleic acid (RNA), yet were oncogenic; but it was impossible for RNA to integrate into DNA. In 1964 Howard Temin proposed the 'DNA provirus hypothesis', suggesting that RSV, an RNA virus, made DNA at some point in its replication cycle: this DNA would make RNA, which in turn went on to make proteins for new viruses. The idea that DNA could be made from RNA ran counter to the 'central dogma', which held that DNA made RNA made protein. In 1970, Temin and David Baltimore announced their independent discoveries of reverse transcriptase, an enzyme which catalyses the conversion of viral RNA to DNA by RSV and other retroviruses. Temin's provirus theory had been proven correct, bringing a unity to the study of oncogenic viruses by suggesting that it is viral DNA which plays such an important role in oncogenesis.

Retroviruses

With the discovery of reverse transcriptase, retroviruses became a popular focus of study, and in 1979 Robert Gallo, later to become famous for his part in the discovery of the human immunodeficiency virus (HIV), discovered the first human retrovirus, human T-cell lymphotropic virus type 1 (HTLV-1).

HTLV-1 is linked to adult T-cell leukaemia/lymphoma (ATLL), and can cause a multiple sclerosis-like illness. The world distribution of HTLV-1 is uneven, with high frequencies of infection in southern Japan, Central Africa and the Caribbean, but a low frequency in Europe (Simmonds,

1998). Transmission occurs from mother to infant via breast milk, by sexual intercourse and by whole blood. However, ATLL is rare: it is estimated there is only a 2%–5% chance of developing ATLL or related neurological disease over an infected individual's lifetime (Gallo, 1995).

Although the closely related retrovirus HTLV-2 has been associated with rare cases of hairy-cell leukaemia, the relationship of HTLV-2 to disease is unclear.

Among the HIV-infected population, patients with AIDS have an increased risk of developing Hodgkin's disease, multiple myeloma, brain cancer and seminoma; it seems that the failure of the immune system to control herpesvirus or other viral infections may contribute to these cancers (Goedert et al, 1998).

Human papillomaviruses

Of the 83 or so human papillomavirus (HPV) types, at least 28 affect the genital tract, where their typical clinical manifestation is as genital warts, or condyloma acuminata (Sonnex, 1998). HPV infection of the genital tract is the commonest sexually transmitted viral infection in the UK. Effective management of such infections is an important public health issue given that certain types of HPV cause cervical cancer and other lower genital cancers; cervical cancer is the commonest genital cancer and causes most cancer-related deaths among women in developing countries (McCance, 1998).

Evidence for an aetiological relationship between HPV infection and cervical cancer came first from sensitive molecular techniques that detected HPV DNA in cervical tumours. There are two classes of genital HPVs: low-risk types are not usually associated with malignancies, whereas high-risk HPVs are. High-risk types, such as HPV-16 and HPV-18, are commonly found in cervical cancers (Lowy et al, 1995). There is a relationship between HPV infection and the development of premalignant lesions in the cervix. These lesions are defined as mild, moderate or severe cervical intra-epithelial neoplasia (CIN 1, CIN 2 and CIN 3 respectively). HPV infection is the most significant risk factor for the development of premalignant and malignant disease of the cervix (Lowy et al, 1995). For example, women with normal cervical smears who harbour HPV type-16 are more than 100 times more likely to develop CIN 3 compared with HPV-negative women (Sonnex, 1998).

Although the UK cervical cancer screening programme saves lives, the Pap smear is prone to variations in sampling and interpretation, and an estimated 5%–30% of abnormalities are missed (Fricker, 1997). ThinPrep 2000, an automated monolayer slide preparation technique, and PAPNET, a computerised reading system, indicate possible directions for cervical screening in the future. The ThinPrep 2000 system allows HPV testing and cytology to be performed on the same sample, and this may be useful for testing women whose smears contain 'atypical squamous cells of undetermined significance'; however, the cost-effectiveness of such techniques is so far undetermined (McCance, 1998).

There is no doubt that the prevention of HPV infection would reduce the number of genital tract cancers. Antiviral therapy has been unsuccessful and it is hoped that vaccination could prevent infection or eliminate established HPV infection or HPV-associated cancer (Galloway, 1998). The success of a canine papillomavirus vaccine and current human clinical trials encourage the hope that a vaccine will soon become part of an overall prevention and treatment strategy, which can be applied in both developed and developing countries.

Herpesviruses

Thirty years ago herpes simplex virus type 2 (HSV-2) was implicated in the aetiology of cervical cancer, an association enhanced by retrospective seroepidemiological studies, which showed a higher prevalence of HSV-2 antibody in cervical cancer patients than in matched controls. However, sexual activity is associated with both genital herpes and cervical cancer, so there may not be any causal link between the two. The idea that HSV-2 caused cervical cancer diminished as evidence implicating HPV increased.

In the late 1950s Denis Burkitt, a Scottish surgeon working in Uganda, began describing tumours of the jaw in African children. He found that Burkitt's lymphoma (BL) had a restricted geographical distribution corresponding to that of hyperendemic malaria, which was determined by climatic conditions favouring malaria-carrying mosquitoes. This suggested the involvement of an infectious agent, and in 1964 at London's Middlesex Hospital, Epstein and Barr, using electron microscopy, discovered the Epstein-Barr virus (EBV) in BL cells. As well as being the cause of infectious mononucleosis (glandular fever), EBV is linked to BL by the following evidence:

- all patients with BL have high concentrations of antibody to EBV
- EBV is present in all BL tumour cells
- most BL tumour cells can be induced to produce EBV
- EBV can transform, or 'immortalise', B lymphocytes *in vitro*, an ability required for any virus causing a B cell lymphoma (Spriggs, 1985)

EBV-associated BL only occurs in those areas where there is hyperendemic malaria (equatorial Africa and New Guinea), making a strong argument for malaria as an important factor in the aetiology of BL. It has been suggested that BL arises in children whose immune systems have been suppressed by malaria since infancy; EBV would find it easier to replicate in children whose immune systems have been thus weakened. It is interesting to note that:

- the incidence of BL has fallen in areas where malaria eradication has been achieved
- the incidence of BL is low among children with the sickle cell trait, which partially protects against malaria (Crawford and Edwards, 1987)

Undifferentiated nasopharyngeal carcinoma (NPC) is a malignant tumour affecting the squamous epithelium of the nasopharynx. In southern China it is the most common cancer of men and the second most common cancer of women.

EBV is linked to undifferentiated NPC by the following evidence:

- EBV DNA is found in the malignant epithelial cells of all biopsy samples
- all of the malignant epithelial cells express a particular EBV protein called Epstein-Barr nuclear antigen
- all sera from undifferentiated NPC patients have high concentrations of EBV antibodies
- EBV can be grown from malignant epithelial cells from NPC

Evidence of family clustering points to a genetic factor in the aetiology of NPC, and environmental factors such as diet and chemical contamination of soil and food may also have a role (Crawford and Edwards, 1987).

Although there is no firm association between cytomegalovirus (CMV) and any human cancer, a recent hypothesis suggests that breast cancer may be caused by late exposure to a common virus; this hypothesis is explored using CMV as a surrogate for a breast cancer virus (Richardson, 1997).

Human herpesvirus type 6 (HHV-6) consists of two related but distinct viruses, HHV-6A and HHV-6B. Studies of a possible relationship between HHV-6 and cancer have focused mainly on lymphoproliferative disorders and, although not conclusive, have found that for some cancers, there is evidence of a degree of association with these viruses (Braun et al, 1997).

Kaposi's sarcoma (KS) is a multifocal tumour found in a high proportion of HIV-infected male homosexuals. There are four clinical categories of KS:

- classic, or Mediterranean
- African endemic
- transplant-associated, or iatrogenic
- epidemic, or AIDS-associated (Braun et al, 1997)

Human herpesvirus type 8 (HHV-8) is linked to KS by the following evidence:

- HHV-8 DNA has been detected in all forms of KS and in about half of blood samples from KS patients, but not from healthy blood donors
- the detection of HHV-8 in the peripheral blood mononuclear cells of asymptomatic HIV-infected patients is predictive for the development of KS
- the detection of HHV-8 in bronchoalveolar lavage fluid is predictive for pulmonary KS (Birley and Schultz, 1997)

However, because HHV-8 can be detected in the blood and semen of individuals who do not have KS (Offerman, 1996), infection with HHV-8 alone does not appear to cause KS.

Hepatitis B and Hepatitis C

The immune system clears most hepatitis B virus (HBV) infections. However, in a proportion of patients HBV may persist as a chronic infection for years. During this time, HBV DNA may integrate into hepatocyte DNA increasing the probability of progression to primary hepatocellular carcinoma (HCC) (Zuckerman and Harrison, 1987).

HCC is one of the 10 commonest cancers in the world, occurring more often in males than in females, with a five-year survival rate of less than 5% (Ince and Wands, 1999). HCC is more prevalent in sub-Saharan Africa and Southeast Asia than in the industrialised countries of the world. There is a relationship between persistent or past HBV infection and the development of HCC, with HCC following the same geographical pattern of distribution as that of persistent HBV infection. In those with persistent HBV infection, the risk of HCC increases by a factor of 100. It is thought that in those areas of the world where HCC is prevalent, the early acquisition of HBV among infants and children and development of a persistent HBV infection are important factors in the development of HCC in later years.

The availability of an effective HBV vaccine means that hepatitis B and HCC are potentially eradicable diseases. The benefits of universal and childhood vaccination programmes have been confirmed by studies in several countries where HBV infection is highly epidemic. These show a marked decline in hepatitis B, chronic hepatitis B and HCC among different populations (Dowdle and Orenstein, 1995; Ince and Wands, 1999).

In addition to HBV, hepatitis C virus (HCV) infection plays an important role in the development of HCC (El-Sherag and Mason, 1999). Persistent HCV infection is an important risk factor for HCC and about 80% of HCV-infected individuals develop a chronic infection. As with HBV, the risk of developing HCC among individuals with chronic HCV infection is 100 times that in uninfected individuals (Ince and Wands, 1999). However, unlike HBV, there is no HCV vaccine, but it is hoped that effective antiviral therapies can be developed which could eradicate HCV infection or prevent its progression to chronic liver disease.

References

Birley, H. D. L., Schultz, T. F. (1997) Kaposi's sarcoma and the new herpesvirus. *Journal of Medical Microbiology*; 46: 6, 433–435.

Braun, D. K., Dominguez, G., Pellett, P. E. (1997) Human herpesvirus 6. *Clinical Microbiology Reviews*; 10: 3, 521–567.

Crawford, D. H., Edwards, J. M. B. (1987) Epstein-Barr virus. In: Zuckerman, A. J., Banatvala, J. E., Pattison, J. R. (eds) *Principles and Practice of Clinical Virology*. Chichester: John Wiley & Sons.

Dowdle, W. R., Orenstein, W. A. (1995) Quest for life-long protection by vaccination. In: Roizman, B. (ed.) *Infectious Diseases in an Age of Change*, Washington: National Academy of Sciences.

El-Sherag, H. B., Mason, A. C. (1999) Rising incidence of hepatocellular carcinoma in the United States. *New England Journal of Medicine*; 340: 10, 745–750.

Fricker, J. (1997) Cervical-cancer screening comes of age-or does it? *Lancet*; 350: 1010.

Gallo, R. G. (1995) A surprising advance in the treatment of viral leukemia. *New England Journal of Medicine*; 332: 26, 1783–1785.

Galloway, D. A. (1998) Is vaccination against papillomavirus a possibility? *Lancet*; 351: suppl. III, 22–24.

Goedert, J. J., Cote, T. R., Virgo, P. et al. for the AIDS-Cancer Match Study Group (1998) Spectrum of AIDS-associated malignant disorders. *Lancet*; 351: 1833–1839.

Ince, N., Wands, J. R. (1999) The increasing incidence of hepatocellular carcinoma. *New England Journal of Medicine*; 340: 10, 798–799.

Krontiris, T. K. (1995) Oncogenes. *New England Journal of Medicine*; 333: 5, 303–306.

Lowy, D. R., Kirnbauer, R., Schiller, J. T. (1995) Genital human papillomavirus infection. In: Roizman, B. (ed.) *Infectious Diseases in an Age of Change*. Washington: National Academy of Sciences.

McCance, D. J. (1998) Human papillomaviruses and cervical cancer. *Journal of Medical Microbiology*; 47: 5, 371–373.

Offerman, M. K. (1996) HHV-8: a new herpesvirus associated with Kaposi's sarcoma. *Trends in Microbiology*; 4: 10, 383–386.

Richardson, A. (1997) Is breast cancer caused by late exposure to a common virus? *Medical Hypotheses*; 4:, 491–497.

Simmonds, P. (1998) Transfusion virology: progress and challenges. *Blood Reviews*; 12: 171–177.

Sonnex, C. (1998) Human papillomavirus infection with particular reference to genital disease. *Journal of Clinical Pathology*; 51: 9, 643–648.

Spriggs, D. R. (1985) Cofactors in disease: Epstein-Barr virus, oncogenes and Burkitt's lymphoma. *Journal of Infectious Diseases*; 151: 5, 977–978.

Zuckerman, A. J., Harrison, T. J. (1987) Hepatitis B virus chronic liver disease and hepatocellular carcinoma. *Postgraduate Medical Journal*; 63: suppl. 2, 13–19.

Appendix 1
Useful addresses

Whilst every effort has been made to ensure accuracy, the publishers cannot vouch for the comprehensiveness of this list and interested readers are advised to consult the *Nursing Times Directory*.

Creutzfeldt-Jakob Disease

Helpline: 01380 720033

Cytomegalovirus

Congenital Cytomegalovirus Association,
c/o Stan and Fay Courtney,
69 The Leasowes,
Ford,
Shrewsbury SY5 9LU
Tel: 01743 850055

Hepatitis

British Liver Trust,
c/o Alison Rogers,
Central House,
Central Avenue,
Ransomes Europark,
Ipswich IP3 9QG
Helpline: 01473 276328; tel: 01473276 326; fax: 01473 276327.
National hepatitis helpline: 0990 100360

Hepatitis C Support Group,
c/o Gabrielle Page,
112 Hunter Avenue,
Shenfield,
Essex CM15 8PG.

Herpes

The Herpesviruses Association,
c/o Marian Nicholson,
41 North Road,
London N7 9DP.
Helpline: 0171 6099061; tel: 0171 6079661

Rubella

National Congenital Rubella Surveillance Programme,
c/o Pat Tookey,
Institute of Child Health,
Department of Epidemiology and Biostatistics,
30 Guildford Street,
London WC1N 1EH
Tel: 0171 2429789, ext. 2604

Appendix 2
Some features of selected human viruses

Virus	Nucleic acid	Illness	Transmission	Incubation period (days)	Laboratory specimens
Rhinovirus (Over 115 types)	RNA	Mainly upper respiratory tract infection (URTI)	Hand-hand, finger–eye, finger–nose, aerosols, fomites	2–3	Nose and throat swab (NTS)
Respiratory syncytial virus	RNA	Bronchiolitis, URTI, febrile fits	Contact with infected droplets and infected fomites	3–5	Nasopharyngeal aspirate (NPA) for rapid diagnosis
Influenzavirus types A and B	RNA	Influenza	Mainly respiratory	1–6	NTS (adult), NPA (child), serum
Human rotavirus	RNA	Diarrhoea (vomiting)	Faecal–oral	1–4	Faeces
Hepatitis A virus	RNA	Hepatitis	Faecal–oral	15–40 mean 25	Serum
Hepatitis B virus	DNA	Hepatitis	Parenteral	30–150 mean 75	Serum
Hepatitis C virus	RNA	Hepatitis	Parenteral	15–120 mean 50	Serum
Varicella zoster virus (VZV)	DNA	Chickenpox Shingles (caused by reactivation of VZV, often years later)	Mainly respiratory	10–21 mean 14	Vesicle fluid or vesicle base swab, serum. Not vesicle crusts

Handwashing is the best simple measure of preventing the spread of viruses in the hospital ward.

Appendix 3 Abbreviations

A	adenine
AHC	acute haemorrhagic conjunctivitis
AIDS	acquired immunodeficiency syndrome
APME	acute post-infectious measles encephalomyelitis
ATLL	adult T-cell leukaemia/lymphoma
AZT	zidovudine, or azidothymidine
BAL	bronchoalveolar lavage
BL	Burkitt's lymphoma
BSE	bovine spongiform encephalopathy
BSI	body substance isolation
C	cytosine
CIN 1	mild cervical intraepithelial neoplasia
CIN 2	moderate cervical intraepithelial neoplasia
CIN 3	severe cervical intraepithelial neoplasia
CJD	Creutzfeldt-Jakob disease
CMI	cell-mediated immunity

CMV	cytomegalovirus
CNS	central nervous system
CPE	cytopathic effect
CSF	cerebrospinal fluid
DNA	deoxyribonucleic acid
DV	diarrhoea and vomiting
EBV	Epstein-Barr virus
EIA	enzyme immunoassay
EKC	epidemic keratoconjunctivitis
EM	electron microscopy
ER	endoplasmic reticulum
EV-70	enterovirus type 70
FITC	fluorescein isothiocyanate
FVS	foetal varicella syndrome
G	guanine
H	haemagglutinin
HAV	hepatitis A virus
HbcAg	hepatitis B core antigen
HbeAg	hepatitis e antigen
HbsAg	hepatitis B surface antigen
HBV	hepatitis B virus
HCC	hepatocellular carcinoma
HCV	hepatitis C virus
HDV	hepatitis delta virus

HEV	hepatitis E virus
HFMD	hand, foot and mouth disease
HHV-6	human herpesvirus type 6
HHV-7	human herpesvirus type 7
HHV-8	human herpesvirus type 8
HIV	human immunodeficiency virus
HPV	human papillomavirus
HSV	herpes simplex virus
HSV-1	herpes simplex virus type 1
HSV-2	herpes simplex virus type 2
HTLV-1	human T-cell lymphotropic virus type 1
HTLV-2	human T-cell lymphotropic virus type 2
HuCV	human calicivirus
Ig	immunoglobulin
IM	infectious mononucleosis
KS	Kaposi's sarcoma
LCR	ligase chain reaction
MCV	molluscum contagiosum virus
MIBE	measles inclusion body encephalitis
MMR	measles, mumps and rubella
mRNA	messenger ribonucleic acid
N	neuraminidase
NDV	Newcastle disease virus
NKs	natural killers

NPA	nasopharyngeal aspirate
NPC	nasopharyngeal carcinoma
NRTI	nucleoside reverse transcriptase inhibitor
NTS	nose and throat swab
nvCJD	new variant Creutzfeldt-Jakob disease
ONS	Office for National Statistics
PCP	*Pneumocystis carinii* pneumonia
PCR	polymerase chain reaction
PIV	parainfluenza virus
PML	progressive multifocal leucoencephalopathy
PTLD	post-transplantation lymphoproliferative disorder
RNA	ribonucleic acid
RSV	respiratory syncytial virus or Rous sarcoma virus
RT	reverse transcriptase
SRSV	small round-structured viruses
SSPE	subacute sclerosing panencephalitis
T	thymine
TSE	transmissible spongiform encephalopathy
U	uracil
UPs	universal precautions
VTM	virus transport medium

Index